8|18

THE RIGHT FIT FORMULA

RTHE IGHT FIT FORMULA

**YOUR PERSONALITY + FAVE FOODS + LIFESTYLE =
THE *ONLY* WEIGHT LOSS PLAN FOR YOU**

CHRISTINE LUSITA, CPT

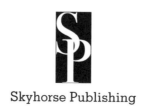

Skyhorse Publishing

Skyhorse Publishing books may be purchased in bulk at special discounts for sales promotion, corporate gifts, fund-raising, or educational purposes. Special editions can also be created to specifications. For details, contact the Special Sales Department, Skyhorse Publishing, 307 West 36th Street, 11th Floor, New York, NY 10018 or info@skyhorsepublishing.com.

Skyhorse and Skyhorse Publishing are registered trademarks of Skyhorse Publishing, Inc., a Delaware corporation.

Visit our website at www.skyhorsepublishing.com.

10 9 8 7 6 5 4 3 2 1

Library of Congress Cataloging-in-Publication Data

Names: Lusita, Christine, author.
Title: The right fit formula : your personality + fave foods + lifestyle =
    the only weight loss plan for you / by Christine Lusita, C.P.T.
Description: New York, NY: Skyhorse Publishing, 2018.
Identifiers: LCCN 2017050973 | ISBN 9781510729759 (hardcover: alk. paper) |
    ISBN 9781510729766 (ebook)
Subjects: LCSH: Weight loss. | Weight loss–Psychological aspects. | Food habits.
Classification: LCC RM222.2 .L77 2018 | DDC 613.2/5–dc23 LC record available at
    https://lccn.loc.gov/2017050973

Cover design by Mona Lin
Cover photograph by mattbeard.com

Print ISBN: 978-1-5107-2975-9
Ebook ISBN: 978-1-5107-2976-6

Printed in the United States of America

To Pauline Terranova, my loving grandmother,
who taught me to live in faith.

Contents

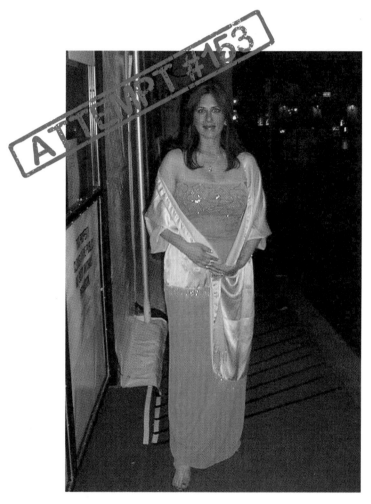

ATTEMPT #153

No doubt I'm about to start diet attempt #153—
miserable much?

Introduction

■■■

Hi! I'm Christine, and I'm a Recovering Yo-Yo Dieter!

EVER SEE THAT CRAZY LADY at the gym, the one who's pumping the StairMaster so hard that you start mentally rehearsing CPR?

That used to be me.

Ever hear of someone who ate only Apple Jacks for three months because it was the easiest way to track calories?

Me again.

I also used to be the woman who wore nothing but black to disguise my belly and worried daily that someone was going to ask if I was pregnant. (They asked. I wasn't.) I would binge-eat peanut butter one day and throw out a whole pot of vegetables the next if I saw one drop of gravy in it. (Yes, "gravy" means "sauce" when you're Italian!)

IN SHORT, I USED TO BE NUTS. For years, I treated my body like an experiment I failed at daily. I hit the cardio equipment like a maniac, obsessed over Jane Fonda tapes, weighed food, drank shakes, ate prepackaged meals, fasted, you name it. And then when I still didn't look like Christy Turlington, I'd park my butt on the couch, get out the ham and cheese sandwiches, and quit. Until I'd hear about the next get-thin-quick fad (and we all know there's no shortage of those) and then start up again "on Monday."

For me, thinness wasn't just a good idea. It was everything. Back then, I believed heart, soul, and mind that if I was thin I would finally feel good about myself, that I would have value, that I would be enough.

I rode that roller coaster a long time before something finally pushed the pause button. One day when I was moaning about how "nothing works" and how hard it was to lose weight, my wise friend Flavio pointed out that the problem wasn't "out there," but in me. "You don't value yourself," he said. "And you can't change what you don't value."

I let that sink in for a moment. It was true: I didn't value my efforts. Ever. I only judged them. I couldn't remember the last time I'd eaten anything with pleasure, taken a run just for fun, or in fact did *anything* that didn't involve a whip at my back. I'd never asked myself: What did I *like*? What did I enjoy, what did I seek out, what motivated me? *Who was I?*

That was the first step on the road of getting healthier. Gradually, and with lots of influences and support, I decided to dial back on the pursuit of skinny and look at my real self, without judgment.

Who was I?

How I Got Real

For starters, I was five-foot-three, small-boned, curvy. (Even at 98 pounds, I knew *Vogue* magazine was never going to come looking for me.)

I liked action. I liked control. I liked leading projects, running with my own ideas. (So why was I working as a secretary?)

I was Italian. I loved food. I ate for holidays, I ate for emotion, I ate because the sun came up. (Why was I torturing myself with Egg Beaters and fake butter?)

I was competitive. I loved the beach and outdoors, but I hated boot camps and team sports. (Why was I doing triple StairMaster sessions?)

Those were some tough "whys." All my life I'd been hearing about workouts and diets that were supposed to be good for me. You can't throw a dart at a newsstand without hitting yet another headline about some magic formula. But each time I "failed," I felt as if *I* were the problem. I knew something had to change, and it wasn't about finding the next gimmick. It was about finding what worked *for me*.

I began carefully listening to myself and, piece by piece, began letting go of yo-yo Christine. I let go of the food that left me feeling deprived. The hamster-wheel workouts. The self-judgment for not being perfect. Even the job I hated. At each step, I worried (and that's another of my traits: I worry!) that I would end up miserable and overweight. But surprisingly, each time I tried something that I kind of liked, that made sense to my mind and felt good to my body, I felt better.

I started my own business—and loved it.

I ran on the beach—and loved it.

I ate my beloved steak and lobster but kept the portions reasonable. And *without feeling miserable and deprived*, I arrived at my best body size and bought clothes that flattered my body instead of hiding it.

Most important, I got happier. That was a new one! Yo-yo Christine was a wreck. When I weighed 100 pounds, I felt anxious and deprived, neurotically counting every calorie. When I weighed 140 pounds, I felt depressed and disgusting.

> **But eventually I learned that self-love didn't come with a number.
> It came through honoring my uniqueness.**

I learned to be brutally honest with myself on what I will or won't do, and I learned to set reasonable goals that inspired me without comparing myself to others. I learned to tackle that tough inner critic that derails all dieters on their weight loss journey. I learned to carve out time for myself without guilt and celebrate my accomplishments. I learned to prioritize and, above all, to value who I am *as I am*.

Today as a diet and fitness coach, I've spent the past 15 years teaching what took me so long to learn: *To manage food and fitness, you first have to manage yourself.* My goal is not to introduce yet another magic formula. My goal is to help you become your best self—your fittest, most balanced, and happiest self. And my goal is to make it *easy*, to make your success a sprint instead of the marathon I've gone through, along with millions of other long-term dieters. In fact, my philosophy for success today can be summed up in four words: Do what feels good!

I've made the mistakes and learned from them. And because I know how hard it is to change, I realized there had to be a system to streamline this process. It *can't* be this hard.

Finding Freedom: I did it, and so can you

In this book, I've created the easiest program possible for permanent, realistic transformation. You'll find the steps you need to reach your goals, the motivation to stay the course, and the support for when your progress derails. This is a precise, no-bullshit program based on your true authenticity—*your* personality and values. Your program will not look like anyone else's. It will pinpoint exactly what fitness and food work *for you.*

Every chapter in this system has been designed to give you freedom: freedom from the diet merry-go-round, from food and workout confusion, and from worrying about setbacks. You'll be given the freedom to be *you*. I call this system the *Right Fit Formula* because it ends the yo-yo dieting cycle, forever. It's about discovering your real self in order to become your *best* self, and being happy while doing it!

Listen, I know I'd probably sell a lot more books if I promised you Gwyneth's abs or Rihanna's legs. But since you probably don't share their genetic makeup or personal chefs, I'm pretty sure you could add that book straight to the top of your Been There, Done That pile.

This book, on the other hand, is one you haven't seen before. It's the culmination of 15 years of working with people exactly like you—people who have no time, tons of stress, and a constant battle with the mirror and scale. I've culled the best of behavioral science, including Acceptance and Commitment Therapy (ACT), widely regarded as the most effective weight loss technique, which focuses on dieters' values, behaviors, and decision making. By combining ACT with mindfulness training, personality profiling, and unique goal-setting techniques, I've created the The Right Fit ID, a one-of-a-kind, solid, and supportive weight loss and lifestyle program. The foundation of the program is to build rhythm, regularity, and routine into your everyday living.

So if you've tried and failed and tried and failed, then please step off the roller coaster for a while and take this journey with me. I've been where you are, I feel you, I *am* you. But I've also found the way through to health and happiness, and I'm so excited to take you there.

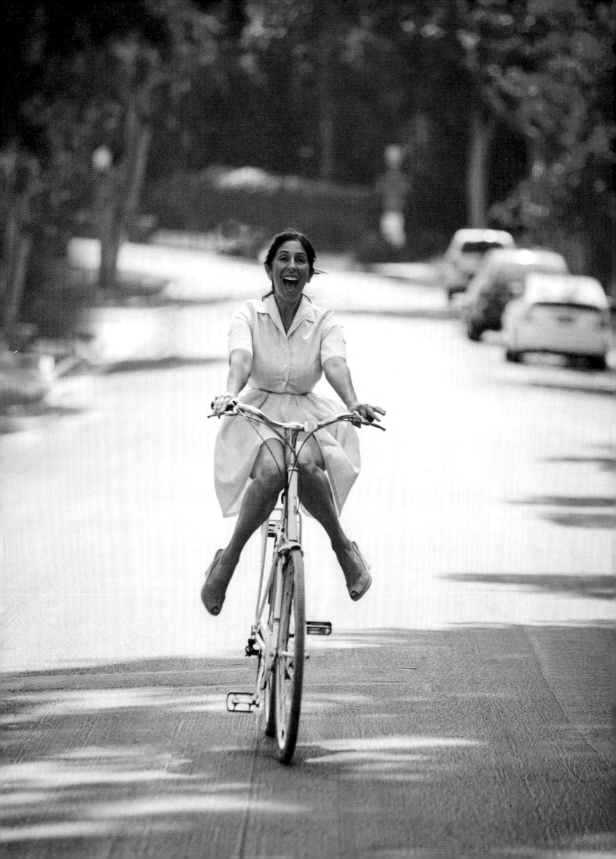

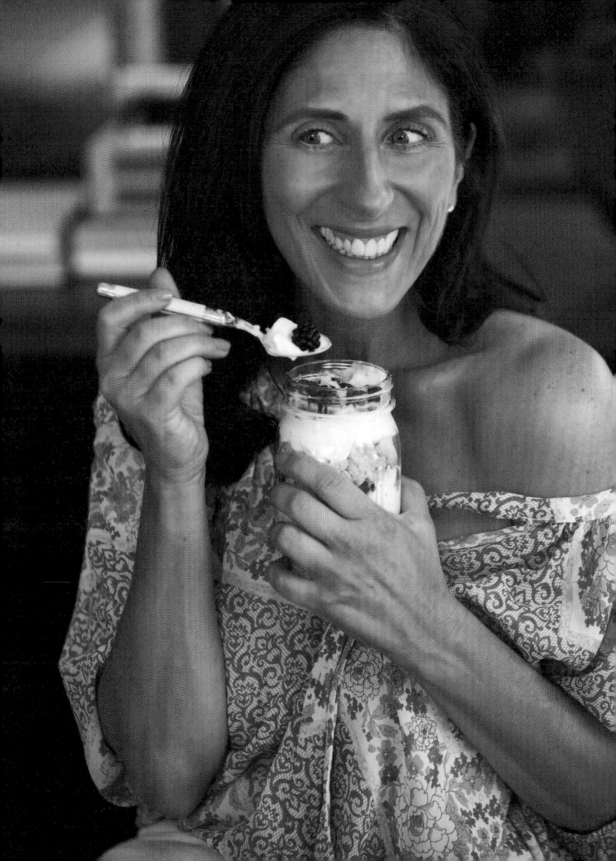

CHAPTER ONE

Stop the Diet Merry-Go-Round! I'm Nauseous, Already

■■■

It's A Mad, Mad, Mad, Mad Diet World

POP QUIZ: Are bananas good or bad? How about potatoes? Beef? Chocolate?

Not sure? Okay, let's try another tack. Is fasting good or bad? How about running? Hot yoga? Weight training?

Here's my point. From the time I was 13, these types of questions ruled my life. I was obsessed with finding *the* answers to losing weight. I couldn't look at food as tasty and nutritious, and I couldn't look at exercise as fun or relaxing. Things were either Good or Bad, and that label changed daily, depending on what I'd read, heard, or seen on TV. Ketchup is bad! Bananas are bad! A hamburger is healthy! A hamburger will kill you! Fast 12 hours a day! Eat six small meals a day!

You can relate, right? After all, this year alone, 1,500 new diet books will be published. That's on top of the "information" in thousands of websites, articles, click-bait, and even the old-fashioned health section of the newspaper. How the heck is a person supposed to sort it out?

I'll tell you the way that *doesn't* work. And that was my old way, which was to try everything. Nutrisystem, Weight Watchers, Zone—name it, and I tried it. It couldn't be that the diets were the problem—didn't they work for those girls on TV? It only made sense that *I* was the problem. So my failure usually took one of these guises:

* **I have no willpower.** Gwyneth Paltrow can eat cookies made with cashew meal—why did I have to go for the Mallomars?

* **I don't have enough time.** I can't go to work, hit the gym, *and* find six ways to prepare kale!

* **I'm exhausted.** *I don't have enough energy.* I can last only 20 minutes on the treadmill—that's not enough to make a difference!

* **I'm lazy.** Eighty-year-old women are running marathons. What's my excuse?

* **This is too hard; I'm never going to get there.** I hired Cindy Crawford's trainer once. He made me do so many lunges that I threw up within the first 10 minutes. Totally my fault, I'm sure.

....

By the time I hit rock bottom with my diet quest, I was overweight, defeated, and completely stressed out. Only when I started "recovering" from repeat dieting, years later, did I realize this fact:

> *It is true that almost every diet plan can be a medically or scientifically successful weight loss path.*

> *But that didn't mean it was my path.*

Among all the diet and fitness books and articles I'd read and followed, there was no resource out there *specifically* geared to Christine. No book or program understood my personality, my lifestyle, and my schedule. I had been trying to plug my complex and unique self into one mismatched diet plan after another. No wonder I wasn't "succeeding."

I "failed" Weight Watchers, for instance, because I obsessed about points and calorie counts. I "failed" Nutrisystem because *I* like to be in control of the food I pick to eat. I "failed" health shakes because I'm a meat-and-potatoes girl, and drinking never felt like eating. It was only when I really got to know myself—my strengths, weaknesses, my be-my-own-boss personality—that I began making choices that made sense to me.

Adios, Egg Beaters

I began taking tiny weight loss steps that worked within my decisive, action-oriented personality. For instance, I knew I hated no-option diet plans. So I began eating consciously and intentionally, choosing food I enjoyed and that felt good in my body. If I felt horrible after eating Egg Beaters, for example, I knew I couldn't sustain a diet of that. If I felt horrible after eating too much pizza, I knew I had to dial that back. Instead of just "eating," I began to really check in, and to educate myself (without going calorie-counting-crazy) about portion size and nutrition.

It was the same with exercise. I began running on the beach because it felt good. But if one day my body felt like walking instead of running, I would tell myself that was okay. Or if I didn't really feel like giving 100 percent, I'd say, fine, do it at 20 percent. Then, if I had more energy (I always did), I'd use it and feel even better. In fact, I found that simply being emotionally flexible (which you'll hear more about) became *the* best strategy for staying consistent.

Over time, each tiny step made me feel better not only physically, but emotionally. During my yo-yo years, I'd set huge, impossible goals, like running five miles after not running in six months. Or not eating bread—one of my favorite foods—for 90 days. Or making sure I ate no more than 1,200 calories in a day. I thought big goals meant that I was action-oriented, a real achiever. But all it really meant was that I was beating myself up if I wasn't perfect. Even when I "made" my goals, it was never enough.

> *By working with who I was, as I was, I managed to step off the dieting merry-go-round for good. And I sympathize with how hard that can seem for the millions of repeat dieters out there.*

NEXT STOP: SANITY

The first step to success, then, isn't to try sorting through the dieting confusion. It's to find out who you are. Knowing your strengths and weaknesses is a game-changer in weight loss. Once you've made that assessment, you'll intuitively connect to habits and effective strategies that will last a lifetime.

The next chapter presents the first and most important step to finding your diet freedom: personal alignment. You'll learn how *The Right Fit Formula* can guide you to your first "aha" moment in knowing which weight loss approach works best for you. I'm excited to point out that this book represents the first time this system has been created for diet and fitness profiling. It's a match.com for your perfect weight loss plan.

The rest of the book will help you explore more sides of your unique style of healthy living. You'll learn about working within your time priorities, your readiness to change, your energy level, and your self-talk.

After many years of coaching and creating customized weight loss and fitness plans, I can say this with confidence: All success is intentional. Weight loss does not happen because the right diet happened to fall out of the sky. It happens because we manage the process, and this book will help you through every single stage.

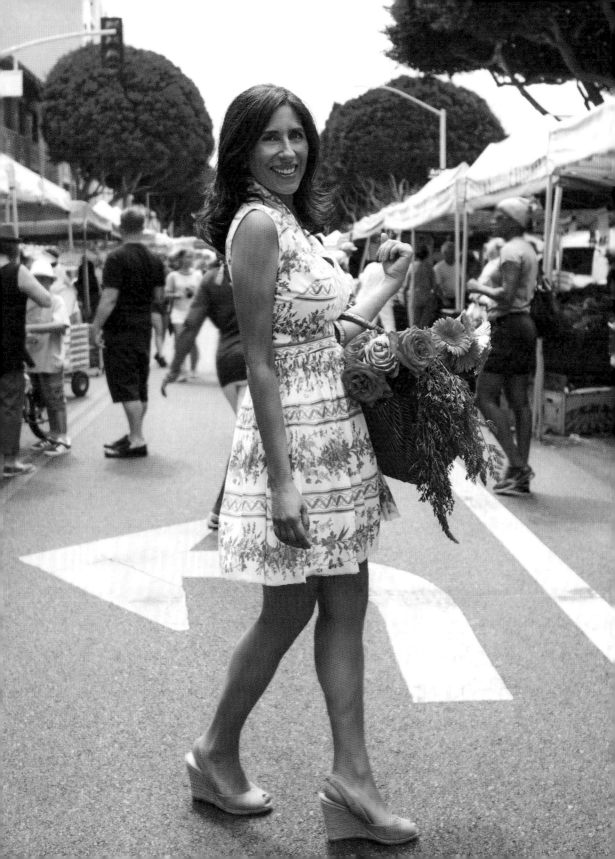

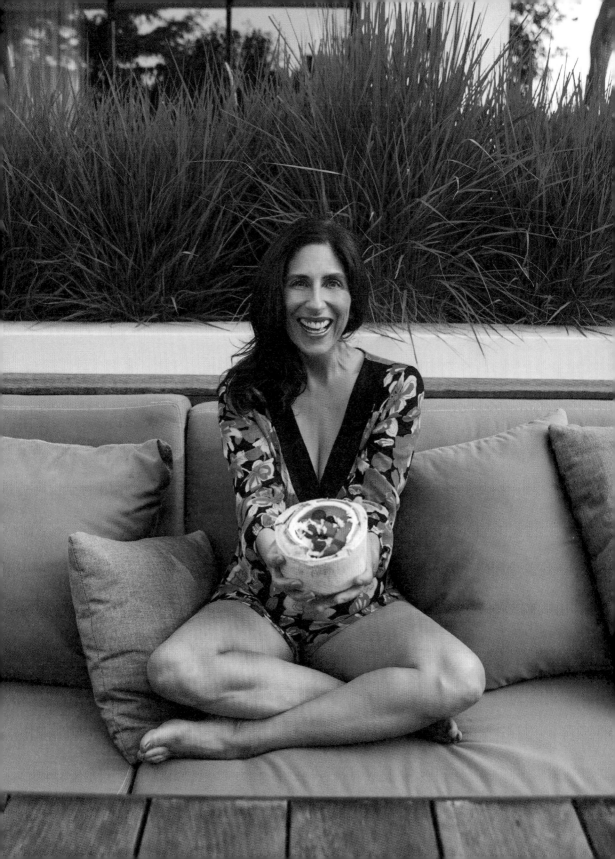

CHAPTER TWO

SWF Seeks Long-Term Relationship w/Diet Sanity

■■■

Repeat Dieting Is like a Lifetime of Bad Dates . . .

YOU START OFF EACH TIME with starry-eyed hope and end up once again lying on your couch with a remote and a bag of Doritos, wondering what the heck is "wrong" with you and whether you'll ever find "the one."

I have two pieces of good news for you.

The first is that choosing the right diet is a whole lot easier than finding a mate. The second is that the key to doing it is right here in these pages.

> *You're about to find that the missing link between your success and repeated diet failure is simply finding the right fit.*

Let's review a couple of facts. This year alone, 1,500 new diet books will be published. Almost all of them are medically and scientifically sound. *But none of them are specific to you.* Not one takes into account your emotional and physical reality. They don't understand your time pressures, your limitations, your strengths and weaknesses. They don't know if you're impulsive or perfectionist, or if you're a workaholic or superanalytical.

And that matters! We all know that most people who attempt to lose weight don't reach their goals, and that most who *do* reach their magic number typically gain the weight back. *That is not their fault.* The vast majority of dieters who "fail" are not lacking in willpower. They are simply mismatched to their weight loss plans. They're pursuing boot camps, spin classes, and Paleo plans based on *who they want to be* instead of who they *authentically are.* And that's the kind of attitude that puts them right back on the repeat-dieting merry-go-round.

More good news. Once you're aligned to a food and workout plan that complements your strengths, you're no longer lying on the couch wondering, "What's wrong with me?" Instead, you're intuitively connecting to habits that will last a lifetime.

Here's an example. Two of my clients, Robert and Yvonne, both wanted to lose weight, and both were completely done in by hamburgers and fries. Neither one could pass an In-N-Out Burger without hyperventilating.

But Robert is a real powerhouse, chairman of an entertainment company. He spends the entire day giving orders and making deals. Subordinates quake when he passes their cubicles. Yvonne, meanwhile, is an engineer. Nothing makes her happier than sitting quietly alone with her diagrams and numbers.

There's no way the same food and fitness program would work for them both. It would be like putting Oprah and Dr. Phil in the same boot camp. Oprah would be dancing her butt off, smiling and trading weight loss tips, while Dr. Phil would be kicking his mat over and glaring down his mustache (*"You're gonna scream in* my *face?"*).

So Yvonne, my analytical client, was delighted with a diet plan that let her calculate calories and experiment with satisfying recipes and food choices. Robert, on the other hand, wanted nothing to do with recipes and food prep. He learned just enough to grill what he liked and hired a chef to prepare healthy meals.

Everyone has a style—a way of being in the world. It's why you choose vanilla or chocolate, Lexus or Infiniti, traditional or modern. And it's how you *should* pick a weight loss or fitness plan—based on your own uniqueness! Knowing who you are helps you understand why certain approaches rub you the wrong way. It helps you trust that inner radar signaling you to beware, to slow down, to avoid trainers, diet plans, and coaches who are not helpful to you.

That's what this chapter, and this book, is about: YOU. Truth is, diets don't succeed—people do.

In this next section, you'll identify your deeply hidden beliefs, personality style, and natural tendencies—all the elements that help you customize your perfect *Right Fit Formula*. No more blind dates with diets!

Remember, there is no right or wrong diet plan. It's just what works for you!

So . . . who are you, anyway?

If you've ever taken a personality test, chances are it was the one developed by psychologists William Moulton Marston and Walter Clarke. Their DiSC program is the gold standard in personality assessment, grouping people by four main categories: Dominant, Influential, Steady, or Conscientious.

It turns out those categories describe my own clients beautifully. In fact, in my many years of practice, I've identified these four types of weight loss clients:

The **LEADER**, the take-charge client who hates being told what to do but goes all-in when something clicks.

The **SOCIALIZER**, who rah-rahs every weight loss idea I throw at her but has just a teeny bit of trouble staying on track because, well, you only live once!

The **SUPPORTER**, the busy, pragmatic soccer mom who hates the idea of anything "trendy" and who says she's running around all the time anyway and doesn't that count?

The **PLANNER**, the disciplined thinker, who loves to discuss the benefits of metabolic conditioning but would rather walk 10 miles than take a Zumba class.

Over the years, I've gotten to know each of these types intimately. I know that a Leader would never end up at the same workout as a Supporter (unless she's leading it!) and that a Socializer will eat very differently than a Planner. Each encounter has helped me understand that nobody loses weight the same way, and that everybody needs a *customized* food and fitness plan that speaks directly to their personalities. That food and fitness plan match is what you're holding in your hands—because for the first time, a coach (that's me!) is going to speak *your* language when it comes to helping you lose weight!

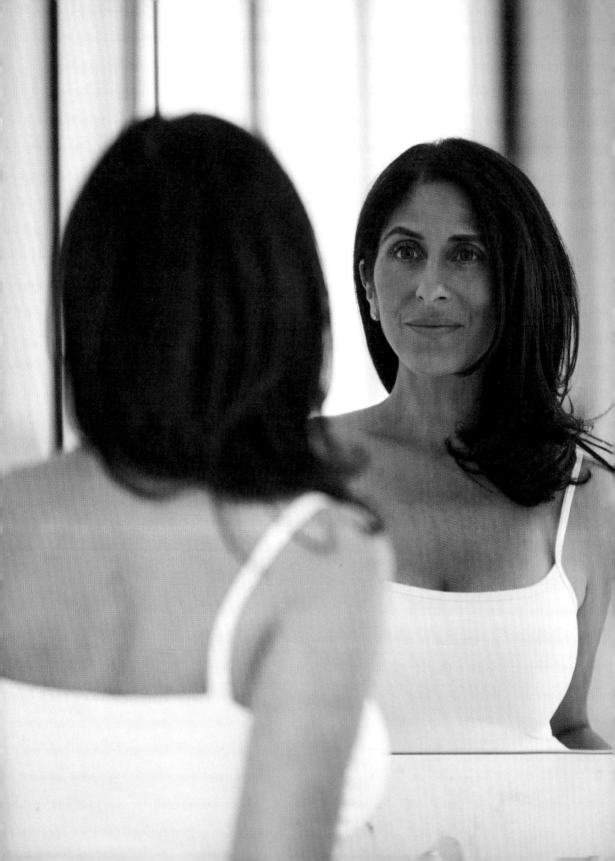

CHAPTER THREE

Let's Get Personal

■■■

Have a Seat. We're About to Get Very Well-Acquainted!

NOW, OF COURSE I don't *know* you. I can't see what you look like, I don't know your age or marital status, and I have no idea how much weight you'd like to lose.

But I do know someone just like you.

That person is in these descriptions below. Take a look at the different personality types and see where you fit best. I'm sure you'll see some of yourself in all these types (humans are pretty complex, after all), but one type will probably speak to you more than the others. That's the personality description that will guide you to your Right Fit ID—the food and fitness plan that will fit you and you alone.

SO LET'S SEE WHO YOU ARE!

The Leader

Also known as: *The Queen*, *The Big Chief*, *The HBIC*, *The Boss*

Leaders are like Robert, my take-charge client. Robert is direct and fast-paced. He sees the big picture and makes fast decisions. Robert can negotiate a million-dollar deal without breaking a sweat, but OMG if he has to balance his checkbook.

If you're a Leader, you are:

- ⋆ **Immediate and decisive.** You lead the meeting and can pick a great idea from 10 losers.

- ⋆ **Always in front.** You don't stand in line, you don't take orders. You were the first to sign up for TSA's PreCheck at the airport.

- ⋆ **Risk-taking.** Nothing delights you more than someone saying, "You can't do that," and proving them wrong.

- ⋆ **Delegating.** If you're a chef, you can't remember the last time you chopped an onion.

- ⋆ **One-of-a-kind.** You follow your own star. No one's going to put Lady Gaga in a corporate pantsuit.

- ⋆ **Willing to act.** People want you sitting in the airplane exit row.

What gets in your way:

- ⋆ **Impatience.** *How much longer do you have to wait in this line?*

- ⋆ **Lack of trust.** If you are a chef, you told that onion-chopper the right way to chop, and you watch him like a hawk.

- ⋆ **Looking before you leap.** Yes, your spouse really will care if you buy that new Audi!

- ⋆ **Highlighting what's wrong, not what's right.** There's a reason subordinates quake around you! Not everything is a problem waiting for you to solve it. Look for the good!

If you hand a Leader a generic food and fitness plan, she will:

Hand it to her assistant.

Pop Culture Leaders: Miranda Priestly in *The Devil Wears Prada*, Rizzo in *Grease*, Samantha Jones in *Sex and the City*, James Bond, Rocky Balboa, Madonna

---

The Socializer

Also known as: *The Cheerleader, The Optimist, The BFF, The Flirt, Miss Congeniality*

Socializers shape their environment with pretty persuasion. Oprah Winfrey is a terrific example: she's warm, open, expressive, an instant pal. If you start feeling great when someone walks in the room, that's a Socializer shedding pixie dust over you.

If you're a Socializer, you are:

* ★ **Persuasive.** You nod when you listen, look everyone in the eye, and get people to perk up their ears when you've got an idea.

* ★ **Charming.** You're the center of the group picture, the one everyone invites to the party.

* ★ **Spontaneous.** You throw a last-minute dinner party, the whole neighborhood shows up, and you're determined to make it fun for all.

* ★ **Optimistic.** You're the Unsinkable Molly Brown, singing on the lifeboat of the Titanic.

* ★ **Empathetic.** Your hugs are famous.

What gets in your way:

* ★ **Disorganization.** Because you can't say no, you need a to-do list for your to-do list.

* ★ **Allergic reaction to detail.** *Couldn't someone else please put together those reports?*

* ★ **Quest for eternal youth.** You're the one still flirting with the young babes or boys after 20 years of marriage.

* ★ **Impulsiveness.** Do you really need that pair of Ferragamo boots?

* ★ **Lack of follow-through.** Something more interesting is always coming down the pike . . .

If you hand a Socializer a generic food and fitness plan, she will:

Enthuse like crazy, swear it's the best, and forget about it in three weeks.

Pop Culture Socializers: Oprah, Tony Robbins, Linda Belcher in *Bob's Burgers*, Ellen Degeneres, Dolly Parton, Jack in *Will and Grace*

The Supporter

Also known as: *The Soccer Mom, The Community Pillar, The Backbone, The Diplomat*

Supporters are quintessential team players. They're calm and centered, the human "pause" button in a heated meeting. Any marriage counselor worth the money is going to have some major Supporter in her.

If you're a Supporter, you are:

* **Accepting and tolerant.** The homeless guy gets as much respect from you as the mayor.
* **Inclusive.** You make sure the quiet student at the back of the room gets to say something.
* **Other-centered.** The whole family knows if you're going to be late for dinner, and you offer to pick up Chinese if it's easier.
* **Diplomatic.** You're the flight attendant keeping the cabin calm.
* **A creature of habit.** The barista has your half-caf skim latte ready before you're at the counter.

What gets in your way:

* **Same-old, same-old.** You've worn ruts in the road between your house and your favorite restaurant.
* **Putting yourself last.** Your "me" time is a hot shower.
* **A why-change attitude.** You've lived with the broken stove for six months because what if someone tries to fix it and makes it worse?

If you hand a Supporter a generic food and fitness plan, she will:

Pretend to consider it, but really, why rock the boat?

Pop Culture Supporters: Charlotte in *Sex and the City*, Michelle Obama, Dr. Oz, Rachel in *Friends*, Mike Brady in *The Brady Bunch*

The Planner

Also known as: *The Scientist, The Perfectionist, The Thinker, The Realist*

Yvonne, our engineer above, is the prototypical Planner. She's soft-spoken, reserved, analytical, and precise. If a Leader decides to go skydiving, she better hope that a Planner packed the parachute!

If you're a Planner, you are:

⋆ **Thorough.** *Consumer Reports* is your favorite magazine.

⋆ **Logical.** As a toddler, you preferred *I am a Bunny* to *Green Eggs and Ham*.

⋆ **Accurate and hard-working.** You make sure you produce at your absolute best, and you expect the same from others.

⋆ **Curious.** Just how does the mono version of "Let It Be" compare to the original Phil Spector production?

⋆ **A lover of detail.** You're the piano tuner, the watchmaker, the root-canal specialist.

What gets in your way:

⋆ **Perfectionism.** It can take a looooong time to get to your "absolute best." Most times, "done" is better than "perfect"!

⋆ **Indecisiveness.** Your stove stays broken because you can't figure out which handyman will do the best job.

⋆ **Opacity.** Nobody knows what you're thinking! Caution and restraint are your operating methods.

If you hand a Planner a generic food and fitness plan, she will:

Check your credentials and conduct her own research to see if it make sense.

Pop Culture Planners: Miranda in *Sex and the City*, Monica in *Friends*, Jerry Seinfield, Katie Couric, Larry David

Uncovering Your Right Fit ID

Yes, I know: Nobody falls neatly into the above categories. Oprah, for instance, has definitely got some Leader mixed in with her Socializer personality. And quintessential Planner accountants can be great at parties.

But chances are you definitely lean in one direction. That direction will determine your Right Fit ID, the food and fitness plan that makes sense to you.

So here's a quick pop quiz to help you narrow it down. Don't worry about whether more than one answer fits or doesn't fit; just pick what sounds most like you. Have fun with it!

When you go to a new restaurant, you like to:
a) Order the chef's special
b) Get input from tablemates so you can share
c) Look for something familiar
d) See what looks like the best value

If you could afford to, you would:
a) Hire a private chef
b) Rent out a trendy restaurant for your birthday party
c) Hire someone to make and pack your kids' lunches
d) Hire the world's top nutritionist to tell you what to eat

At dinnertime, you'll often find yourself:
a) At a business meeting
b) Out with friends
c) With family
d) At your desk

If you don't have the time to cook, you usually:
a) Go to a drive-thru
b) Call a friend and go out
c) Find something you froze last week
d) Drink a protein shake

When you open your refrigerator, you see:
a) Whatever the housekeeper put in there
b) Lots of wine and snacks
c) Leftovers
d) Nine containers of yogurt (they were on sale)

The workout routine that makes the most sense to you might be:
a) Racquetball
b) Zumba classes
c) Walking the dog
d) Golf

The last time you blew off your workout, you were probably:
a) On a plane
b) Slightly hung over
c) Dealing with a to-do list
d) On a deadline

You would rather eat nails than:
a) Join a boot camp
b) Swim laps
c) Take a trapeze class
d) Play pick-up basketball

On the other hand, you might not mind:
a) Having your own gym
b) Trying beach volleyball
c) A next-door yoga studio
d) Taking up martial arts

Your best reason for getting fit is to:
a) Avoid a heart attack
b) Look great
c) De-stress
d) Maintain optimal health

IF YOU PICKED MOSTLY A'S:

Your Right Fit ID is *LEADER*. You want immediate results, and you don't want to fool around with too much prepping, shopping, or calorie counting. If you could, you'd hire a chef and trainer and build a gym just so you could get fitness over with as quickly as possible.

For you, a food and fitness plan might include:

* ⋆ Simple, easy food plans
* ⋆ Flexible, portable meals (the drive-thru is the Leader's Waterloo!)
* ⋆ One-on-one competitive sports, like running and racquetball
* ⋆ Adrenaline-rush workouts, like sprinting or singles tennis

And it would definitely not include:

* ⋆ Complicated recipes and kitchen prep
* ⋆ Lengthy discussions about fitness details
* ⋆ Boot camp trainers who get in your face
* ⋆ Group classes

Great diet matches for you include: Mediterranean, Paleo, Biggest Loser Diet or the Flex-itarian Diet, all of which offer plenty of options and simple plates.

. . . .

IF YOU PICKED MOSTLY B'S:

Your Right Fit ID is *SOCIALIZER*. You want to work out in social settings and talk, talk, talk about diet, food, and what's working and what isn't. If it were up to you, every meal would be celebrated on Instagram and every workout would end with a wine-and-cheese mixer.

For you, a food and fitness plan might include:

* ⋆ Some type of group support to share eating plans and results
* ⋆ Fun workouts, such as dance; or social team sports, such as volleyball or softball
* ⋆ A cooking club or recipe swap

And it would definitely not include:

- ★ Solo sporting ventures, like lap swimming or track
- ★ YouTube workouts (unless you're the one filming them!)
- ★ Detailed calorie counting and food weighing

Great diet matches for you include: Weight Watchers, The Wild Diet, The Spark Solution Diet, or Jenny Craig, all of which offer plenty of support, interaction, and community.

. . . .

IF YOU PICKED MOSTLY C'S:

Your Right Fit ID is ***SUPPORTER***. You're all about family time and obligations, and you probably feel guilty even for scheduling workout time! You'll have to be convinced that fitness is worth your time and effort.

So for you, a food and fitness plan might include:

- ★ **Accountability.** No wacka-doodie workouts. You want something with a proven track record.

- ★ **Convenience.** Drive across town to break a sweat? *Please.* You have a life!

- ★ **Familiarity.** You don't care about that skinny gal in *People* magazine. You want to know how your hairdresser got back into her high-school jeans.

- ★ **Numbers.** You want equipment that tracks your progress and calories. When you hit 30 minutes or 300 calories, ding! You're outta there!

- ★ **A firm schedule!** If it can't happen at the same time every day, it's probably not going to happen.

And it would definitely not include:

- ★ Anything trendy or kooky-sounding
- ★ Foods and supplements that come only from certain stores or websites
- ★ Workouts that require special equipment or too much time

Great diet matches for you include: Mayo Clinic, Volumetrics, Nutrisystem, and the Zone diet, all of which are all moderate and measured.

. . . .

———

IF YOU PICKED MOSTLY D'S:

Your Right Fit ID is *PLANNER*. You're a label reader, a calorie counter, a data cruncher. You know—or you plan to know—what glucose does to blood sugar and how gluten is processed in the colon.

For your logical, analytical personality, the right food and fitness plan would include:

* ★ Anything with well-researched and proven methodologies. If there's science behind it, you won't mind combining certain foods or cooking in precise methods.
* ★ Equipment that provides benchmarks and feedback.
* ★ Journaling to track your progress.
* ★ Slow-paced workouts—martial arts, lap swimming, pilates—that include skill-builiding and precision.

And it would definitely not include:

* ★ Trendy diets or workout groups.
* ★ Zumba classes, dance, aerobics, and other "just have fun" workouts.
* ★ Fast-paced trainers who push for action.

Great diet matches for you include: The Dash Diet, The Whole 30, TLC, and The Macrobiotic Diet, all of which include plenty of logic, science, and realistic approaches to weight loss.

HEY, WE'RE JUST GETTING STARTED!

Keep in mind that this is just your entry point to your personal *Right Fit Formula*. Granted, if you love the idea of checking out a trendy diet, go for it! But if you want to really dial into a customized plan that you can follow for life, stick around. The following pages will give you everything you need.

Meanwhile, I bet you're relieved to know a little something about why your past yo-yo cycles didn't work out! You can forgive yourself, Planner types, for never joining the company softball team. It's okay, Supporter friends, that you gave up on Jenny Craig. Those programs are complete mismatches for your personality. And you Leaders: Stop kicking yourself for "failing" Weight Watchers and Nutrisystem. It's okay that you're not into group fitness and that you prefer to choose your own food! (That's why I became a coach—as a Leader, I'm great at knowing what others can do, and guiding them on how to do it!)

Knowing your personality is the first step to matching yourself to your optimal plan for losing weight and getting fit. From here, you can blaze a path to success that's as unique and resilient as you are.

We'll be talking much more about food and fitness matches throughout the book. But before we get there, let's take your "readiness" pulse to find out how prepared you are to tackle a new food and fitness plan. The best time to try something new is at the peak of excitement. If you're like me, the clarity you now have is a nice little turbo thrust to keep going. Stay with me, and you'll end your journey with a customized weight loss plan. Diet freedom is only steps away!

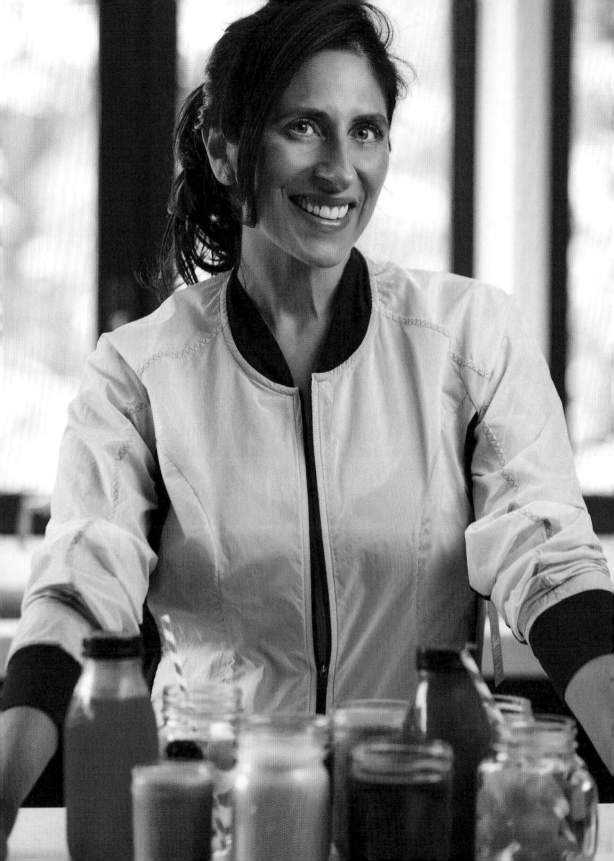

CHAPTER FOUR

The Cure for "I'll-Start-Monday" Syndrome

■ ■ ■

You Can't Hurry Love . . . or Change . . . or Weight Loss!

I HAVE A FRIEND who decided that she was going to quit sugar. Forever. So the day before she quit, she said good-bye to her sugar by loading up on brownies and ice cream and Frappuccinos.

Sound familiar?

Hey, we all have the I'll-Start-Monday Syndrome. For instance, every year I made a New Year's resolution to lose weight. Every year I failed. Because change does not happen on a certain date, not even January 1. Change is a process. It takes time. It requires balance and rewards.

Here are three truths about change, which reveal why my well-meaning friend was back on sugar within a week.

Truth Number One: Positive change happens organically.

Most of us approach dieting as if jumping into an unheated pool: with gritted teeth and grim determination. It doesn't really matter if we "know" it's the right thing to do. All we know is that it doesn't feel very good, and the bigger the dieting change we make, the less good it feels.

Author James Clear, the habit-change guru, tells us that *any* change, positive or negative, sets us up for resistance. And, he writes, "Resistance is proportionate to the size and speed of change, not to whether it's favorable or unfavorable." That's because nature—particularly human nature—is geared toward stability. With apologies to Science 101, a body at rest tends to stay at rest, and if that same body is forced into cross-training every day, it's going to want to double-down on TV time.

So the best way—and often the only way—to sustain positive change is to do it *as it feels right*. If you're cutting out sugar, do it one packet at a time until *that* becomes the new normal. Baby steps!

Truth Number Two: Positive change happens slowly.

It's common wisdom that a new habit takes at least 21 days to form. It's also common wisdom that reaching that 21st day is very challenging, and for these reasons:

★ **We're not seeing immediate results.** If you're pulling back on sugar, for instance, those excess pounds aren't exactly puddling onto the floor. One pound of weight is 3,500 calories. You have to give up that delicious morning muffin *every day* for a week to move the scale. It takes a while for the perceived benefit to catch up with the perceived effort.

★ **We are feeling immediate pain.** After days of dieting, most of us may not look thinner, but we sure feel grumpier. Even after all that sacrifice, your stomach still sits in your lap, the sun is not shining brighter, and the world is not the oyster you thought it would be. So why not have that extra bite of cake, given that the miracles you'd hoped for have not materialized?

★ **We haven't prepared ourselves for change.** To create new habits, we need support, accountability, rewards, positive self-talk and a flexible plan. It's unlikely that gritted teeth alone will get anyone through 21 days.

Truth Number Three: Positive change requires honest motivation.

Clarity is critical for sustained weight loss. *Why* you want to change will inform your commitment to change. If you want to look like Christy Turlington (Repeat Dieter Christine raises her hand), your chance of real change is zero. If you want to lose weight for your boyfriend, your chance is only slightly better. It's only when your motivation comes from an authentic place (*I'm uncomfortable, I'm short of breath, and I know I look and feel much better at a different size*) that you can really stay the course when things get rocky.

So now that we've faced the hard truths about change, let's get back to you and what you're ready to transform in your life. Remember, there are no "shoulds" in this program! You'll discover for yourself your own way and pace for change.

The Five Stages of Change

Whether it's about getting married, changing jobs, or losing weight, everyone goes through five stages of change, as identified by behavioral psychologist James Prochaska. Change starts with pre-contemplation, where you're just kinda, sorta starting to think about making a move. And it ends with maintenance, where the change is now an established habit, part of your everyday life.

THE FIVE STAGES

Stage 1: Pre-contemplation

Stage 2: Contemplation

Stage 3: Preparation

Stage 4: Action

Stage 5: Maintenance

It's safe to say that many dieters want to go straight to Stage 5, where they envision themselves happily eating salads and saluting admirers as they run on the beach. But while I can't shortcut the stages for you, I can help you move through them with purpose and energy. So let's jump in—because in my pool, the water is perfect for you.

Stage 1: Pre-Contemplation

At first, you might be tempted to skip this stage. After all, you're reading this book. Doesn't that already mean you're contemplating change?

Answer: not exactly. Most people who "fail" at change do so because they haven't honestly answered four critical questions:

1) What do you really want to change?

2) How important is this change?

3) How confident are you that you can make this change?

4) What does it mean if you don't make this change?

To demonstrate how this works, I'm going to interview my former self, Repeat Dieter Christine, who wanted to drop 25 pounds so she could look like Christy Turlington.

On a scale of 1 to 10, how important is this?
RDC: Definitely a 10. I have to lose this weight!

On a scale of 1 to 10, how confident are you that you can make this change?
RDC: I'm super motivated! However, I've tried about 30 times already, so I'm maybe a 6 that this time I'll do it?

What does it mean if you don't reach this goal?
RDC: Well . . . I don't know. I guess I'll just be the same as I am now. I mean, I really would love to look like her . . .

Now I'll recap an interview with Anne, one of my clients who also wanted to lose 25 pounds.

On a scale of 1 to 10, how important is this?
Anne: A 10. My doctor told me I'm prediabetic and that I might need knee surgery if I don't lose some weight.

On a scale of 1 to 10, how confident are you that you can make this change?
Anne: An 8. I've been thinking this through, and while it would be great to lose 40 pounds, I feel I will really see benefits at 25. So I'm going there for now.

What does it mean if you don't reach this goal?
Anne: Not reaching it is unacceptable. It would mean more doctors and discomfort, and I really want to stay active and keep playing tennis.

It's pretty clear which dieter was likely to move through the stages of change. Anne really wanted change. She was prepared for Stage 2, Contemplation, in which she would start planning her weight loss program. But Repeat Dieter Christine only *wished* she could lose weight. Because she didn't really value her goal, she was unlikely to commit to making it happen.

So spend a few minutes right now thinking over your own priorities. What do you really want to change, and why? Be honest about ranking yourself. If you score your desires at 5 or below, you might be wishing for change rather than really wanting it. You've spent enough time chasing impossible dreams: make sure your desire for change is important and that you're confident in pursuing it. If what you want isn't really alive for you, you'll be stuck forever at Stage 1.

Pre-Contemplation Analysis

What do you want to change?

_____

On a scale of 1 to 10, how important is this?

not at all   1   2   3   4   5   6   7   8   9   10   very

On a scale of 1 to 10, how confident are you that you can commit to this?

not at all   1   2   3   4   5   6   7   8   9   10   very

What would it mean in your life if you don't make this change?

_____

_____

_____

What would it mean in your life if you do make this change?

_____

_____

_____

How happy are you with the way things are now?

_____

_____

_____

Would making this change create more positives in your life?

_____

_____

_____

I want to describe the moment when I, Repeat Dieter Christine, finally turned serious about losing weight. It was when I stood naked in front of a mirror and asked myself, "What would my life be like if I stayed exactly the way I am, with all my habits and behaviors currently in place?" Instantly I knew I was eating so much sugar that diabetes was on the horizon, as well as depression and isolation. And that was when I knew I had reached Stage 2.

Stage 2: Contemplation

Here's the stage of change in which *wishing* becomes *wanting*. Once you've reached Contemplation, you *know* you want to lose weight. So at this stage, you'll weigh the Pros and Cons of creating the space, will, and energy for that change.

At first, it's probably a lot easier to come up with Cons than with Pros. Here are a few typical ones:

* I don't have the time or energy.

* I don't think it will be fun. It will just be hard work.

* Nobody really cares what I look like.

* I'm too old/young/heavy/unathletic/sedentary to make big changes in my life.

* Holidays are coming up and I should wait.

* I don't have money for trainers/gyms/equipment.

* Etc., etc.

Even the Pros can be problematic. You may think you want change for external reasons, like these:

* ✱ I want to have *her* booty.
* ✱ I want to win my ex back.
* ✱ I'm tired of being jealous of everyone.
* ✱ Etc., etc.

To move through this stage, you need internal motivation. When you compare yourself to others, you devalue yourself; you're telling yourself you're not okay as you are. And believe me, it's very hard to care about changing or improving something you don't value!

Sometimes, of course, external motivation can get the job done, at least for a while. Many of us can kick off those 10 pounds for that wedding or class reunion. Celebrities work very hard to avoid appearing in a "Check out the Muffin Top!" photo gallery. But to go for the long haul, fitness and weight loss need to be part of your core value system.

I can't say this often enough: **VALUE EQUALS EFFORT**. When you know, inside and out, that you are worth the time and effort to get healthy, then you'll do the work of getting healthy. Suddenly, the Cons (the time, the disruption, the expenditure of energy) begin to look a lot less problematic.

So if you're in this stage, spend a few moments really checking in on your process, making sure that you're ready to change for the long haul. Get honest and dig deep!

Contemplation Analysis

What positives do you envision for making this change? Create a list of Pros.

_____

_____

_____

Which of those Pros involve comparing yourself or meeting someone else's wants?

_____

_____

_____

Rank each Pro on a scale of 1 to 10, with 10 being "very important."
Add up the numbers.

_____

_____

_____

Now list what you think will get in the way of your weight loss program (Cons).

_____

_____

_____

Rank each Con on a scale of 1 to 10, with 10 being "very problematic."
Add up those numbers.

_____

_____

_____

Compare your rankings.

Now list whatever strengths you bring to your weight loss challenge. These might include resilience, patience, determination, family support, or anything else that will help in your quest.

_____

_____

_____

Rank each strength on a scale of 1 to 10, with 10 being "very helpful." Add up the numbers, and subtract half that amount from the Cons number.

_____

_____

_____

Now compare your rankings again.

If the Pros come from your core values, and they outrank your Cons, congratulations! You're ready to move forward.

Stage 3: Preparation

At this stage of the game, you're putting your program in motion. You know losing weight is truly a priority for you. You have a core belief that fitness is essential to a balanced and happier life. But now you need to get from "here" to "there."

In Preparation, you'll polish up your strengths and knock out the Cons that get in the way of a healthier you. By the time you're done, putting your plan in action will be a natural next step, not a white-knuckle ordeal.

My client Amy is a good example. She'd been carrying 10 extra pounds for years and felt she was no longer able to keep up with her beloved biking group. But she believed her age was a big Con. She'd been gaining fat and slowing down since menopause and couldn't see how that could change. *And* she didn't want to give up her favorite foods, like bagels.

Fortunately, Amy had a lot of strengths in her favor. She was competitive, realistic, and very motivated to stay active. Together we tested out her Cons. While it's true that weight loss is tougher past menopause, Amy's real issue was that her body had settled into a routine and plateaued. She needed to challenge her body by adding core-strengthening exercise and giving her legs some recovery time. We also switched up her eating so that she could enjoy her bagels *before* a ride, thereby getting a carbohydrate boost for energy. By cracking open her routine, Amy rode more, felt better, and shed pounds.

So at this juncture, you too can move forward by just looking at what you're currently doing and how you can modify it. Throughout the book you'll see tons of ideas for solid preparation, including carving out time, boosting energy, and defeating your inner critic. Right now, here are a few pro tips on how to get started:

Preparation Checklist

☐ **Journal.** Keep a food, time, and exercise log for a few weeks, detailing the way you live your life now.

In my journal, I noticed that I would like to cut back time spent on:

_____

And increase time spent on:

_____

☐ **Explore.** Grab diet plans and workout ideas where you find them. Lay them out on a table and see which ones speak to your personality and lifestyle.

It would be fun to try:

_____

☐ **Shop.** Buy new sneakers. Find fun playlists. Check out farmer's markets and the outer edges of your local grocery store (avoid the aisles, where all the processed food lives). Take note of anything that looks tasty and healthy. Get some pots, pans, and dishes that will make cooking a pleasure.

It would be fun to have:

_____

☐ **Find resources.** Find cookbooks that speak to health and fitness. Seek advice from fit friends and coaches. Check out apps that help you stay focused on your goals.

Five resources I liked:

1) _____

2) _____

3) _____

4) _____

5) _____

Five good pieces of advice:

1) _____

2) _____

3) _____

4) _____

5) _____

☐ **Collaborate.** See if some of your friends want to join your weight loss journey. Or find a Facebook group that can provide tips and accountability.

I wouldn't mind being accountable to:

_____

☐ **Clean up.** I'm a big believer in purging anything that robs you of precious time and energy. (More about that in Chapter 7.) Clearing space makes room for positive change.

Five things in my life/home/office that don't serve me:

1) _____

2) _____

3) _____

4) _____

5) _____

☐ **Build your confidence.** Remember, losing weight is not about turning your life upside-down. It's about working with who you are, where you are. So go at your own pace—but keep going!

Stage 4: Action

Some might think of this step as work. I think of it as play. Now that you've carved out some time, grabbed some ideas, and gained some confidence, you get to explore. You get to try recipes, workouts, and potential new habits and see which ones make sense to your mind and feel good to your body. This is where you really get to check in on your intuition and notice how it feels to do, eat, or practice something new.

Again, it's not about turning your life around. In fact, it's not even about turning your life 90 degrees. It's about moving the needle one tick at a time. Here's how.

Easy Action Steps

☐ **Pick one thing.** It's common wisdom that the more you try to change at once, the less you'll stick with any change at all. A study on ABC News recently pointed out that if you try to change just one habit in your life, you have an 85 percent shot of sticking with it. If you change two habits at once, the success rate drops to 33 percent. So don't try to, say, give up lattes and wine, if you have a habit of both, in a day. Give up one and let yourself have the other, at least until you stop missing your taboo treat. Or keep your taboo treat and create a new habit of, say, 30 minutes of exercise.

List five small things you would like to change to reach your goal. Pick one and commit to it for a week.

1) _____

2) _____

3) _____

4) _____

5) _____

☐ **Start on the path of least resistance.** When I started exercising—in an intuitive, sensible way, that is—I knew I had to keep the bar really, really low. I couldn't stand the thought of "failing" once again. So I decided I would just walk around the block. That's it. And when that became a habit, I started to walk two blocks. Then I might run a block and walk a block. I simply made it impossible to tell myself, "Nope. Not up to that today." That was a game-changer.

What is the easiest way for you to make the change you selected?

_____

_____

_____

What would be the desired final outcome for that change?

_____

_____

_____

(Example: Your desired change is to cut back on your four-day-a-week mocha chip Frappuccino habit. Step One might be giving yourself a Starbucks budget—say, $45 for one month. Step Two might be cutting that budget back $5 per month until your habit is down to, say, one tall Frapp per week, no whip.)

☐ **Play Curious George.** Look around for workouts that sound like they might be . . . fun! Kickboxing, spin classes, yoga-Pilates, ballet, tap dancing, roller skating—exercise options abound in this fitness-conscious world. If you commit to trying something new once a week or every two weeks, who knows what new positive habits you might just adopt and love!

List five activities you would like to try. Commit to trying one for two weeks.

1) _____

2) _____

3) _____

4) _____

5) _____

☐ **Cut yourself some slack.** As I've said before, emotional flexibility is everything when it comes to sticking with your weight loss plan. If you don't feel like giving 100 percent on a given day, tell yourself that you'll give 50 percent. You'll probably be surprised at how much you really can give.

Keep a journal for two weeks of how you feel before and after you exercise. Then answer the following:

How do I generally feel before I work out, on a scale of 1 to 10?

Blah   1   2   3   4   5   6   7   8   9   10   Amazing

How do I generally feel after I work out, on a scale of 1 to 10?

Blah   1   2   3   4   5   6   7   8   9   10   Amazing

Note your average energy level, on a scale of 1 to 10.

No energy   1   2   3   4   5   6   7   8   9   10   Totally pumped

☐ **Just do it!** Ironically, thinking about exercise can be tougher than doing it. Motivation follows action, not the other way around. As a friend of mine likes to say, "The hardest part about milking a cow is putting on your coat." Once you've stepped on the treadmill or even just shown up at the gym, you've already done the hard part. Just take the next step!

Here's something else I tell myself when I don't feel like taking action:

> *Would I rather spend one hour doing whatever I'm avoiding,*
> *or 23 hours kicking myself because I didn't?*

That always gets my butt out of the chair.

List five supportive things you can say to yourself when you don't feel like working out.

1) _____

2) _____

3) _____

4) _____

5) _____

☐ **Adjust as needed.** Say you decided to do your workouts early in the morning. If you find you've got no morning energy, switch it up! Try exercising after work, or take a run during your lunch hour. The point is, you'll never stick with a plan if you keep fighting yourself to do it. It's okay to drop that trainer you don't like; trainers know that not everyone is a match. And if you hate eating Paleo style, try something else. Each time you attempt something new, even if you hate it, you learn more about what works for you and what doesn't.

List five weight loss techniques you tried that did not work for you.

1) _____

2) _____

3) _____

4) _____

5) _____

To the best of your ability, list reasons why these techniques felt like a mismatch.

1) _____

2) _____

3) _____

4) _____

5) _____

Now list what you liked about those techniques, if anything.

1) _____

2) _____

3) _____

4) _____

5) _____

How might you adjust these techniques to make them work for you? Alternatively, what other choices might you make instead of these?

1) _____

2) _____

3) _____

4) _____

5) _____

☐ **Celebrate!** Tell yourself you rock for putting in an extra five minutes on the elliptical. Admire your flatter stomach. Flex a bicep or two. We've all spent way too much time pinching flab and looking for butt sag. This is the time to acknowledge all the things you're doing right, however small you think they may be. If you put skim milk in your coffee today instead of half-and-half, I think you deserve a high-five. Don't you?

List five things you did today that were good choices for you.

1) _____

2) _____

3) _____

4) _____

5) _____

List five easy rewards you can give yourself when you complete something challenging. (Examples: Play one game of solitaire, fist-bump your mirror, spend five minutes on your favorite blog, play a favorite song.)

1) _____

2) _____

3) _____

4) _____

5) _____

Stage 5: Maintenance

At last! Here we are at the end of the rainbow, where you're happily eating salad and saluting admirers as you run on the beach. Just as you imagined.

Wait, what? That's not what's happening?

Here's the final truth about change: The credits never roll. Every day, you really do have to make a choice to keep doing the work that keeps you healthy—or not. The fact is, and I really hate to say this, salad is never going to taste as good as ice cream. And even if you eat salad all day every day, I'm pretty sure you still won't look like the cover of *Elle* magazine.

But I have two pieces of good news for you.

One: At Stage 5, you really look and feel sooooo much better than at Stage 1. Seriously. If you've come this far, that is a given.

Two: At this stage, making good choices really isn't so tough. Little by little, your healthy choices are becoming positive rituals. Just like brushing your teeth and washing your hair, the right diet and workout are becoming a daily routine that your body really wants.

Let me tell you about the time I quit smoking. It was tough. I was not one of those people who could cut back a little at a time, and I wasn't one of those people who could just throw the pack away. Because if I threw it away, I'd eventually buy a pack so I could have just one more. And of course I'd hate to waste all the others in there!

So what worked for me was putting one cigarette in a drawer in my house. Every day, I could choose to smoke it or not. And every day, I simply chose not to smoke it. If I really wanted it, it would be there tomorrow. Knowing that I could choose made me feel as if I were in control, not the cigarette.

In the same way, choosing to work out and stay on track every day isn't always going to be easy. You're going to crave treats, you're going to get bored, and you're going to have setbacks. But *you* can maintain control and stay consistent. Here's how.

Keep it simple. If you're in a setback, just do something physical. Anything. Stand up and stretch if you're stuck working at your desk. Walk the dog. Don't punish yourself because you're not getting in that hour of cardio; congratulate yourself for doing what you can.

Moving your body has two positive results: it gets you out of your head, and it creates an experience. Years from now, when you're thinking back on your life, you'll remember the things you did, not the things you wanted or wished for. So for the sake of helping out your future self, get moving!

Change it up. Particularly for Supporter personalities, plain old boredom can push you right off the weight loss wagon. It's the same old run, the same old treadmill, the same old yoga sequence.

Boredom saps energy and motivation, so don't wait before exploring options. Make it a monthly habit to check out a different gym or workout routine. Or simply add variety to what you're doing already. If you're a runner, for instance, try trail running, or sprinting, or intervals. If you love your boot camp, try substituting a dance class once a week.

Consistency gets results, but variety gets you excited. Variety is satiety!

Create recovery time. In yoga, every posture has a counterposture. For every forward fold, there's a back bend. For every spinal twist in one direction, there's a twist in another. And every session ends with the most important posture of all: savasana, or complete letting go.

That can feel almost like a cheat for those of us who are always "doing." It's counterintuitive. When we spend a precious hour on workout time, we want to see something for it: a tighter butt, a flatter tummy, Michelle Obama arms. You're not going to "see" anything from stretching or meditating or, heaven forbid, resting. But you will *feel* something. You'll feel renewed!

And I'm here to tell you that recovery is crucial to maintenance. My client Amy, for instance, had essentially burned out her leg muscles from constant cycling, and she had upper body problems, such as back pain, from a lack of core strength. *She needed to rest those legs.* By building in recovery time, her legs came back stronger than ever, and she could focus on creating more balance in her upper body.

Recovery also keeps your stress level down—and stress is the number-one reason we reach for the cookies. Every time you're in *active recovery*—i.e., not flopped in front of the tube for five hours—your mind comes to peace and your body is stronger and refreshed.

You'll find many more maintenance techniques throughout the book. Keep checking in with yourself as you reach this stage: You'll maximize your results and minimize your setbacks.

....

Maintenance Analysis

What happens in your life that gets in the way of working out or eating well?

_____

_____

_____

How much of the above is under your control?

_____

_____

_____

What are your top five reasons for blowing off a workout or going off your food plan?

1) _____

2) _____

3) _____

4) _____

5) _____

What positive messages can you give yourself to keep going?

_____

_____

_____

List five easy-peasy ways you can get physical when you're not in your usual workout mode.

1) _____

2) _____

3) _____

4) _____

5) _____

List five ways you can switch up whatever workout you're currently doing.

1) _____

2) _____

3) _____

4) _____

5) _____

List five new workout ideas you might like to try.

1) _____

2) _____

3) _____

4) _____

5) _____

What can you do for five minutes every day just for yourself?

_____

_____

_____

Which of the following interests you as a technique for active recovery?

* Meditation
* Mindfulness
* Stretching class
* Yoga
* Message
* Solo walk or hike (no phone!)

WHEW! THAT WAS A LOT TO TAKE IN!

I hear you, friend. You've just discovered that change is not as simple as "Open Sesame" or "Abracadabra." But hang in there! Remember, I'm all about flexibility, freedom, and choice. In the coming chapters, you'll explore lots of options for finding the time, space, energy, and motivation to change. Go at your own pace and choose what makes sense to your personality, lifestyle, and values. It's progress, not perfection! So turn the page and let's figure out how to deal with one of your biggest lifestyle sticklers (and mine): creating more time!

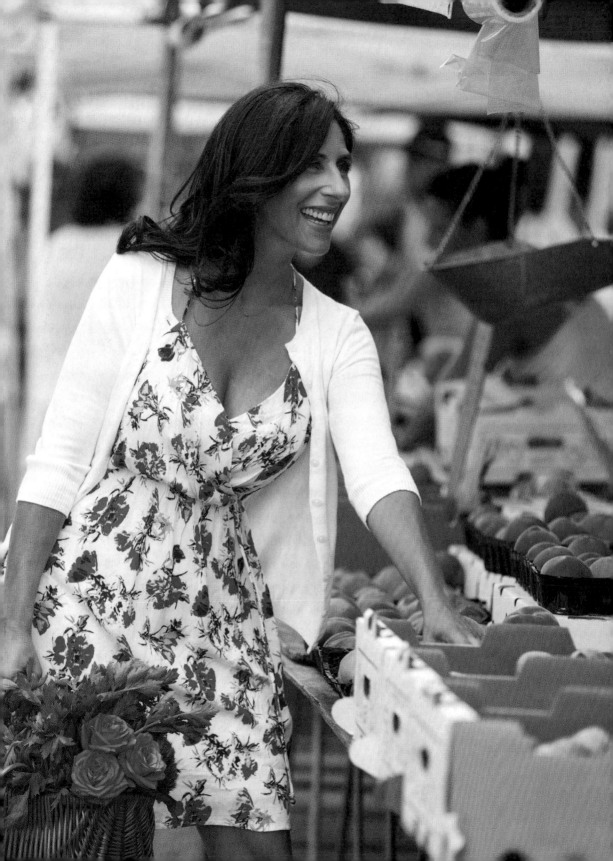

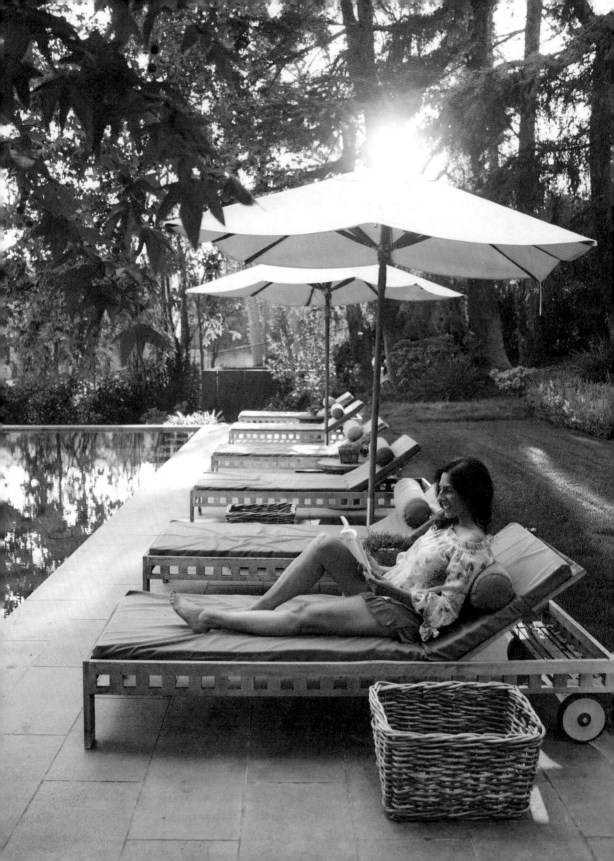

CHAPTER FIVE

Oh Yes, You
DO Have Time!

■■■

Are you the Tomorrow Girl?

THE ONE WHO SWEARS THAT next week is always a better time than right now? "Sorry, no time." "Can't. I'm swamped." "Wish I could. Not right now."

I hear you. And believe me, I used to say that stuff every day. I never had *enough* time! We live in an overachieving world, and nobody's handing out prizes for taking it easy. But I've learned that time is like money. If you don't track it, you never know where it goes. And when you *do* track it, it's a game-changer. As I became more connected to my needs and values—instead of my endless to-do list—I found my time opening up, creating more space for the healthy habits that made sense to me. I even had down time!

So this chapter is about making more time for you, right now. It's about making sure that you have a place in your crazy day for habits that complement your big-picture goals. We're not talking about doing things faster or sacrificing sleep. We're talking about *effectiveness*. When your priority is you, you are time's master.

Urgent vs. Important

Time is *the biggest* challenge for anyone who wants to make real change, particularly when it comes to losing weight. When your day is spent putting out one fire after another—the carpool, the meeting, the report deadline—you can't help but feel there's no time for you. Going to the gym? Forget it. Chopping up vegetables for a healthy salad? Not happening. At the end of a long day, you're going to reach, again, for that nice glass of wine (I deserve it!). And then, of course, the cheese and crackers and the couch are *right there . . .*

But think about this the next time you're having one of those five-alarm days. It's one of my favorite quotes from President Dwight Eisenhower: *What is urgent is seldom important, and what is important is seldom urgent.*

In other words, it's not necessarily time that prevents you from making positive change. It's choice.

Let me tell you about the two executives I use to work with. One arrived at the office an hour before anyone else and was inevitably the last to leave the building. The other walked in at 9:00 on the dot and left at 5:00 on the dot. You'd think that Executive A probably got a lot more done than Executive B. And you'd be wrong. Executive B was more productive than anyone I'd ever seen. Decisions were made and carried out. Meetings were on time and involved everyone's ideas. Reports were approved and moved on. And when Executive B left at 5:00, her briefcase was empty. She was off to watch her kid's soccer game.

That's not time management; that's *choice* management. Executive B had her eye on the prize—family time—so she wasn't going to spend 10 minutes of her workday scrolling through sneakers on Zappos!

It's interesting, though, how so many of us are more like Executive A. With every intention of being "productive," we still can't imagine how it's 5:00 already, we're wiped out, and we haven't really gotten anything done. Our demanding schedules tell us we're *alive*—but are we really living?

I don't want to spend a lot of time on *why* we live in a constant tailspin. For some of us, downtime is just plain uncomfortable, and running around feels better than sitting around. For others, filling up the calendar feels validating: *I'm needed!* Some of us fear that if we aren't pulling our weight, we'll be left behind, like Pete Best at the Beatles reunion. And some of us are procrastinators, spinning through Internet click-bait so we can avoid finishing that project. We all have our reasons for having too much on the plate, and if that's your constant refrain, you might want to soul-search a bit on what all that busy-ness means to you.

But I suspect that many of us are simply not focused on *us*. We haven't set up a schedule that includes the things that are *important but not urgent*—such as relaxation, exercise, and health. After all, if your priority is becoming your best self, shouldn't your best self be in charge of your schedule? Shouldn't you include *me* time in your daily life?

So let's take a look at what's really happening in your own way-too-busy day. Then I'll share with you what I've learned about carving out more time for *you* and you alone.

The 24-Hour Countdown Time Audit Tool

When you actually track your time, you gain clarity. You become aware of where your time goes, and you automatically make more time for your true priorities.

For instance, let me ask you right now how much TV you think you watch in a day. If you're like me, you probably say, "Oh, an hour or two. But really, I'm not a TV person." And yet, A.C. Nielsen, the television-monitoring company, says the average American watches *four hours* per day. To which I say: "Well, not *me!* Oh, yeah, I did watch that movie the other night . . . and of course I watch the news . . . and I binged on *Breaking Bad* for a while . . ." Sound familiar?

My point is this: Few of us actually know the time costs of our daily routines. And that knowledge is key in helping us make better choices.

So I've designed this tool to help you identify what you do in a day, hour by hour. First, I'd like you to estimate how much time you *think* you spend on the following daily activities:

Sleeping	_____
Grooming (showering, etc.)	_____
Eating/preparing meals	_____
Commuting	_____
Working	_____
TV/social media	_____
Family/friends time	_____

Now, spend a day *tracking* each of those activities. By the end of the day, your list might look like this:

Sleeping	*7 hours*
Grooming (showering, etc.)	*1 hour*
Eating/preparing meals	*1.5 hours*
Commuting/working	*9 hours*
TV/social media	*1.5 hours*
Family time	*2 hours*
Total time:	*22 hours*

Those are the actual numbers from my client Emily, a mother of two and a CEO of a Fortune 100 company. Note that at the end of her 24-hour period, Emily had two hours left in her workday! That's 10 free hours a week, plus weekends—enough for a part-time job!

I know what you're thinking: Emily's list didn't include all those errands a person needs to run. What about doctor appointments, movie dates, visits with friends? *What about laundry?*

Relax. My point is this: It's easy to chew up those extra hours running out for milk, or polishing doorknobs, or talking to your neighbor. But if you're making *you* a priority, then even a Fortune 100 executive has time to squeeze in 30 minutes to sweat. Or to schedule a class, take up a hobby, or do something else that will support her best self.

So now take your own inventory with the Time Audit tool below. Be honest! If you find you're spending a couple hours a day doing things in your "Other" category (running to Starbucks, playing computer solitaire, researching Jennifer Aniston's pregnancy status), I'm going to show you how to switch things up and honor your priorities. I want you to end each day knowing you've done something you *loved* and honored what was really important to you. What else is time for?

Now it's your turn.

Your 24-Hour Time Audit

Hours spent:

Sleeping	_____
Grooming (showering, etc.)	_____
Eating/preparing meals	_____
Commuting	_____
Working	_____
TV/social media	_____
Family/friends time	_____
Other	_____

What to Do When Time Doesn't Pay

If you've been humbled by the amount of "wasted" time in your Time Audit, fear not. You're just three steps away from making your time pay off as never before.

Step One: Create a dream schedule.

We all have a list of things we'd do *if only we had time.* Maybe it's volunteering. Or surfing. Or working on that startup clothing line or joining that hot yoga class.

Think about your own "if only" list, and then try reverse-engineering your 24-Hour Time Audit Tool. In other words, create a dream schedule in which you build in time for the choices that matter in your life and cut back on the ones that don't. Let your imagination go wild and don't judge yourself!

Emily, for instance, not only wanted to lose weight, she wanted to work on a script idea that had been on a back burner for years. In her dream schedule, she decided her day would look like this:

Sleeping	*8 hours*
Grooming (showering, etc.)	*1 hour*
Eating/preparing meals	*1.5 hour*
Commuting/working	*6 hours*
TV/social media	*1 hour*
Family time	*3 hours*
Exercise/relax/self-care	*1 hour*
Work on script	*2–3 hours*
Total time:	*23–24 hours*

Your dream schedule:

Sleeping	_____
Grooming	_____
Eating/preparing meals	_____
Commuting/working	_____
TV/social media	_____
Family time	_____
Exercise/relax/self-care	_____
Passion project	_____
Total time	_____

Step Two: Create your preferred schedule

A preferred schedule, of course, would be a hybrid of an actual schedule and a dream schedule. In Emily's case, the preferred schedule *had to* include all her work time—a fact that was naturally discouraging (who wouldn't love to cut back office hours?). But by choosing to delegate some chores and by cutting back on social media, Emily created a schedule that included choices that mattered to her:

Sleeping	*7 hours*
Grooming (showering, etc.)	*1 hour*
Eating/preparing meals	*1 hour*
Commuting/working	*9 hours*
TV/social media	*1 hour*
Family time	*2 hours*
Exercise/relax/self-care	*1 hour*
Work on script	*1 hour*
Total time:	*23–24 hours*

Now she was ready to master her day!

Your preferred schedule:

Sleeping
Grooming
Eating/preparing meals
Commuting/working
TV/social media
Family time
Exercise/relax/self-care
Passion project

Step Three: Create your Top-Three List

You know that to-do list you write at the start of the day? I'm going to ask you to add three items to it, right at the top. Those would be three things you can accomplish that day to support your personal values, goals, and objectives.

Only you know what those three items would be! (Head to the previous chapter if you want some direction on identifying your deepest values.) Meanwhile, I'm going to suggest your Top Three List include these categories:

Self-care. For healthy and authentic living, self-care is not optional. On your list, schedule a workout, a meditation, a hike, a bubble bath, a massage . . . whatever relaxes and recharges. Only when you're rested, healthy, and serene can you live your best life and be your best for others.

Passion. Most of us with a "someday" project—Emily's script, for instance—feel it can't get done unless a magical chunk of time descends like a spaceship from Mars. Trust me—even five minutes a day can push the needle forward. Whether it's stamp collecting, animal rescue, or art history, your passion deserves your attention, daily!

A personal goal. Once you've set a goal (Chapter 8), you've got to keep moving toward the finish line. If you plan to lose 10 pounds, your to-do list might include a meal prep and/or workout. If you want to run a nine-minute mile, your list might include steps for making it happen, even if it's just researching sneakers. Whatever you can do, do today to keep from losing precious momentum.

Your top-three list:

1) _____

2) _____

3) _____

Now pick that "one thing."

This idea is straight from author Gary Keller, founder of Keller Williams, the world's largest franchise real estate company. In his best seller *The One Thing,* Keller suggests "choosing *one* item from your list and making it a top priority." This one simple, powerful concept allows you to focus on and master what matters most.

Choosing "one thing" is especially important when you're just beginning a weight loss program. Ask yourself: *What's that one thing you can do today to support your priority?* Maybe you'll throw out your junk food. Maybe you'll crank up the speed on the treadmill. Every day, pick that one thing that means the most and get 'er done!

My one thing:_____

Urgent vs. Important, Revisited

Now that you know what your optimal day looks like, there's just one teeny challenge left. How do you stay on track? How do you keep from sliding back to the dark side, to the Land of Distractions and Time Sucks? How do you keep your schedule from looking like a page out of John Madden's playbook?

First, take a tip from Executive B: When you're working on your have-tos, work smarter. The quicker you knock the "musts" off your list, the more time you have for the things you love. Remember, it's not time management, it's choice management.

So:

Ditch the distractions. While you're doing your "musts," do not peek at your email. Turn off Instagram, Twitter-feed pings, and Facebook announcements. And no phone. Yup, I said it. No phone. And yesss, you will survive.

Block your time. Give yourself a solid, focused 30 to 60 minutes of undistracted work. Try these two tips from time-management gurus: One, do short bursts of intense work followed by short stretches of recovery (from Tony Schwartz and Jim Loehr in *The Power of Full Engagement*). And two, shorten your deadline and tighten up your schedule so that you'll increase your focus (from Tim Ferriss in *The 4-Hour Workweek*). Focus = productivity!

Take a break. This means making a cup of tea, walking around the room, stretching, folding the laundry, doing a set of pushups, or taking 10 simple breaths at your desk. *This does not mean you get your phone back!* Sorry! Each time you check your email or watch a Kardashian on Instagram, you not only clutter your focus, you create what time-optimization guru Cal Newport calls "cognitive residue." In short, you fill your head with info-gunk that can take up to 20 minutes to clear. Could five minutes of Kardashians rob *you* of an hour of focused work time? Don't take a chance. Get up and stretch!

Have Yourself a Better Time!

I mean that literally. Here are some final tips for building in habits that sneak more time into your schedule.

Schedule your social media time. Give yourself two social media breaks a day, and make them short, please. Mine are two minutes at lunchtime and two minutes at the end of the day. I think of them as minirewards for maximizing my productivity.

Dedicate your workout time. Make it the same time, at least three days a week. Pen it in as if it were grocery shopping, laundry, or any other must-do task. This accomplishes two things: First, it makes your workout a routine, and that improves your chances of getting it done. Plus, when you go off track, a routine is what gets you back on the right path. Second, when your workout is scheduled, you don't waste energy during the day trying to figure out when to fit it in.

Your best workout time is what works for *you*. People with night energy sometimes prefer an afterwork workout, discharging all their stress of the day. Others prefer an early start: Mornings are the time least likely to be interrupted or need rescheduling. Plus, early-morning workouts accomplish what Mark Twain called "eating the frog." His quote: "If you eat a live frog in the morning, nothing worse will happen to you the rest of the day!"

Build in time rewards. I have a friend who loves computer solitaire. She's particularly vulnerable whenever there are a few minutes of free time and the laptop is *right there*. How does she deal? She has to earn it. She won't play a game unless she's knocked something off her to-do list. And then, *just one game*. Result: Productivity, baby!

Remember that every minute counts. It's a message that bears repeating: Just a few minutes a day spent on *important, not urgent* can make a huge difference in living your best life. If you don't have an hour to call your best friend, spend five minutes sending an email with photos. If you'll "never" get to that quilt project, keep the sewing machine at hand and jump in for five minutes at a time. If you really can't squeeze in that workout, put on some Salt-N-Pepa and jump rope for five minutes! True fact: there will *never* be the perfect moment. Grab what time you have, and enjoy the results.

Here's the final takeaway. When it comes to time, you have three choices. One, you can wish for more of it, which is the equivalent of wishing for X-ray vision and an invisibility cape. Two, you can fritter it away with a gossip scoop here and a Candy Crush game there. Or three, you can master it. You can turn that hunk of marble of a day into a pile of rock chips—or into a statue of David. Your *choice*!

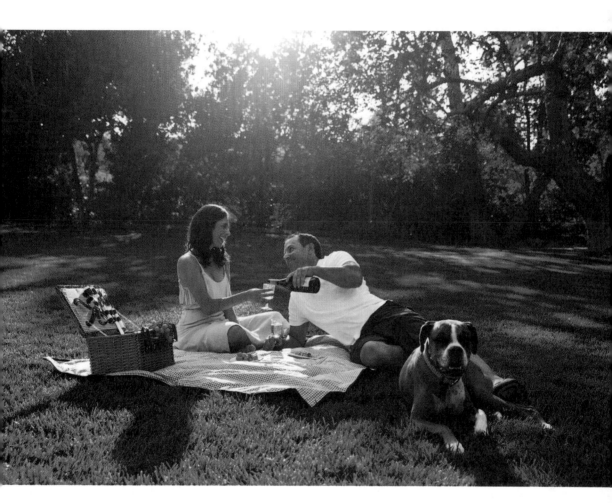

EXCUSES, EXCUSES

Yep, everybody's got a reason why positive change gets shoved to the bottom of the daily inbox. *They* say it's because they don't have time for that workout or that meal prep. *I* say it's because they're not making the best choices. See which excuses sound like *your* excuses, and then let's talk.

The Leader says: My trainer couldn't make it last month, and now I'm too booked up to fit him back in. Things are crazy at the office!

Christine responds: Don't forget about your 15-pound goal by Christmas! And you know that when you exercise you're more productive. Why don't you walk on the treadmill while you're reading the trades? Start there, and we'll start working your trainer in during that time.

The Socializer says: You know I love exercising! And I'll really miss it while I'm showing my cousins around town this week, but once they're gone I'll definitely—oh, wait, that's when I've signed up to go to that music festival (yikes, better start booking a hotel). But after that, *for sure.*

Christine responds: I know you have an intention to sweat every day, so no problem! I'd be delighted to include your cousins in your workout time, and they'll love that new coffee place down the street afterward. Be sure to wear your Fitbit at the music festival; dancing counts!

The Supporter says: Work out? Okay, as in when? My kids come first, the dog gets lonely, and that fancy gym is way too expensive. Besides, I run around all day and burn off plenty.

Christine responds: Since you walk the dog every morning right after dropping the kids at the bus, why don't you take these weights with you? I'll show you easy ways to make that walk more productive, and you won't lose a minute from your schedule. And let's remember how "me" time is a priority for you. If you combine some errands today, you'll buy 20 minutes to relax and meditate.

The Planner says: I was fully committed to going on that bike ride, but my bike shoes were muddy and I can't record a ride log wearing street shoes, can I? So I did crosswords instead.

Christine responds: Remember that "done" is better than "perfect." You've chosen to make your health a priority, and isn't it better to end the day having accomplished your ride instead of your crossword?

What's *your* excuse?

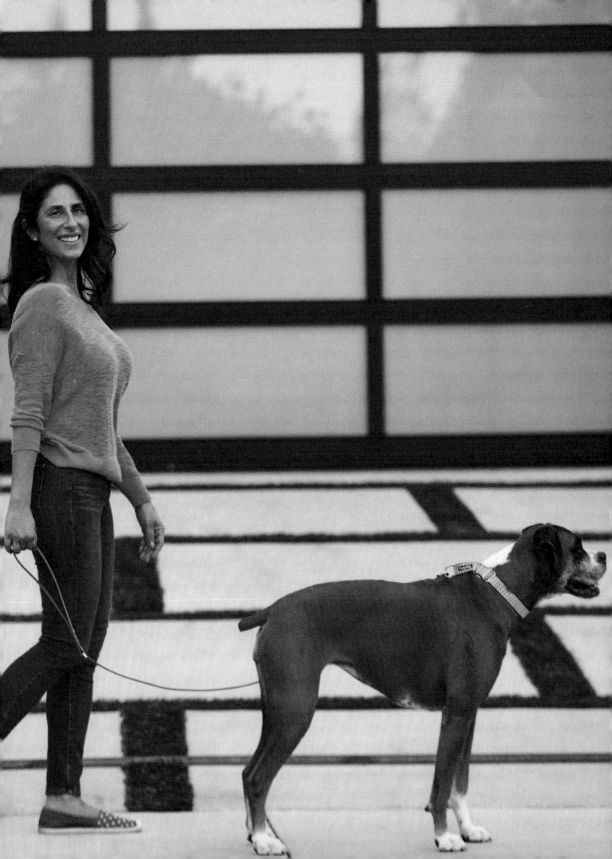

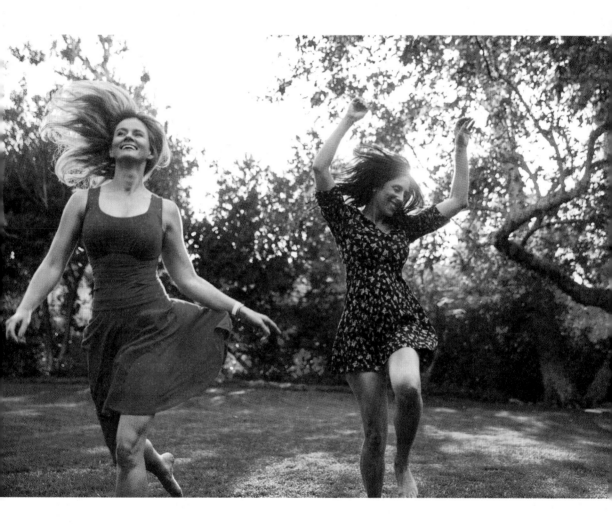

CHAPTER SIX

Energy: How to Make More of It, STAT!

■ ■ ■

Decisions, Decisions: Couch or Treadmill?

I'M THE FIRST TO ADMIT IT: I'm a high-energy person. But for years, I lived in a state of perpetual drain. My life was one have-to after another, and I couldn't even brush my teeth without mentally running through my list. Sleep? Forget it. I spent my pillow time completely in my head, strategizing about tomorrow.

Today's lifestyles are excellent energy drainers. Facebook alone can suck you dry in no time. Add in a few annoying phone calls, an unfinished to-do list, a couple of grouchy kids, and a school board meeting—you're fried and heading straight to the drive-thru!

Can you relate?

As a coach, I've found that *energy* is at the crux of all diet-and-exercise success or failure. You may have great intentions to go for that walk, prep your meal for the next day, or sign up for that workout class, but you'll never get there when you spend too much energy on tasks that rattle you or that aren't in line with your priorities. If you're a quiet Planner who just had to spend the day hosting an office party, you're a zombie. If you're a Leader forced to sit down with a pile of paperwork, someone will have to peel you off the desk. And when you get up, I know exactly where you're going—straight to the Cinnabon counter!

And that's another reason why we're all in an energy crisis. Because this is the 21st century, most of our energy drains are mental, not physical. In its way, an hour in traffic is as draining as an hour pushing a plow, but it's the kind of drain that craves a glass of wine instead of a well-deserved rest. Which means that at the end of a typical modern day, you're exhausted, you're reaching for the bag of cookies and the remote, *and* you're kicking yourself for being "lazy"! You can't win!

When you're in a state of perpetual drain, it's hard to see a way out. In *The Power of Full Engagement*, Tony Schwartz writes that "energy is the fundamental source of all positive action," but it doesn't feel that way when *your* energy is spent wiping peanut-butter smudges off your kid's dresser or looking up your ex on Facebook. So how do you use your energy effectively? How do you put yourself into forward motion instead of a perpetual tailspin?

Well, the solution is not found in a can of Red Bull.

It's found in balance.

You need to expend enough energy to feel strong and competent and in control, and you need enough restoration to feel serene and ready for action.

So in this chapter we're going to take a closer look at what blocks your energy and gives you easy ways to renew it. Don't settle for survival mentality, running on fumes while chasing your to-do list. Aim to *thrive,* to spend your energy on the things that feed your spirit. You're worth it!

Where does the energy go?

First, you have to know where you spend your energy. Here's why:

Energy is also like money. If you don't track it, you never know how or where it gets spent, and you're always at risk of losing it. If you spend it wisely, you reap benefits and have something to show for it: a healthy life, a completed marathon, a finished book, a happy heart.

Your most valuable asset is your attention. Your attention is what you *can* control—and where you spend your attention is where you spend your energy. If you focus on actions that mean something to you, you automatically have more energy. And believe me, the energy shots that come from *within* are a whole lot more effective than the ones you buy at 7–11!

Schwartz said, "To maintain a powerful pulse in our lives, we must learn to how to rhythmically spend and renew energy." The strategies below will help you do just that. They'll help you close the gap between who you are and who you want to be.

So let's get started. Take a look at the Time Audit you created for yourself in the previous chapter. You'll see fairly clearly how your day—and your energy—is divided into four main categories:

1) Work
2) Family
3) Rest/Recovery
4) Self-Care

Now try putting those categories into a pie chart, basing it on energy instead of time.

Before you do, one note: Self-care doesn't mean energy spent on Facebook binges or other procrastination habits. It means energy spent doing those things that actively restore you, like knitting, cooking for pleasure, or (hint, hint) exercise. (If you argue that Facebook or Instagram really does restore your energy, we need to talk.)

Take your energy audit:

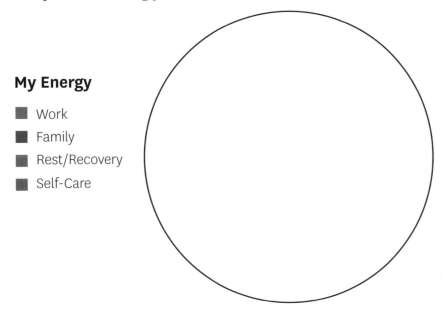

My Energy

- Work
- Family
- Rest/Recovery
- Self-Care

I'm going to go out on a limb here—just take a wild stab—and assume that self-care, *real* self-care—gets just the ittiest-bittiest piece of your energy pie. In fact, I bet that it's barely a sliver next to that giant blob called "Work," and if you have kids, "Family." And that Rest/Recovery category could use some beefing up, too. Any chance I'm right? You. Are. Not. Alone. We don't live in a society that rewards us for *resting* and *recovering*. We live in one that says extra hours at the office make us relevant!

So now the only question is: how do we reslice the pie? Simple: it's a matter of adding and subtracting. By which I *do not* mean adding in TV time while subtracting your to-do list. I mean adding *restoration* and subtracting *energy blockers*.

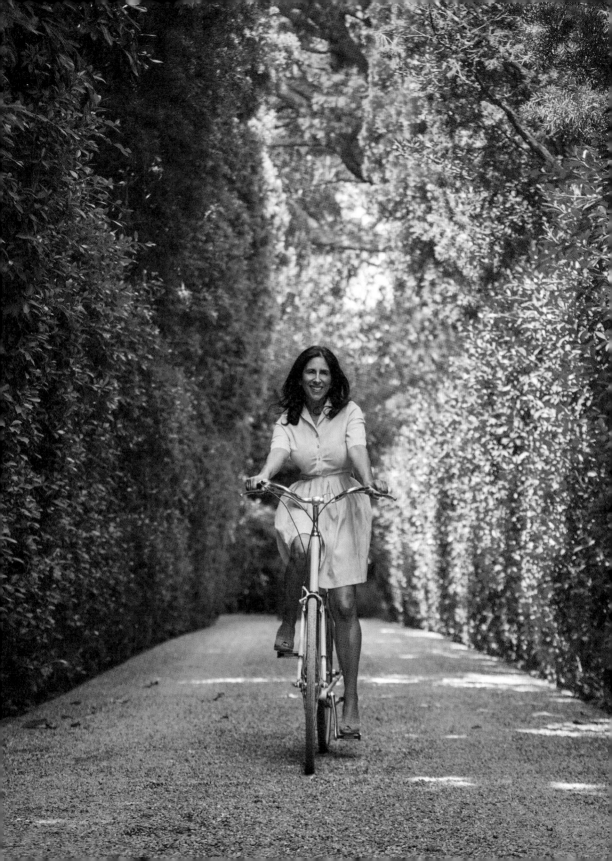

Here's how to start.

Know your enemy! Meet the top 8 Energy Blockers

If you're a typical repeat dieter, you know these guys *very* well. Heck, you may even be BFF's! They're the Energy Blockers that interrupt your best intentions the way your favorite telemarketer interrupts your dinner. See if these sound familiar:

Blocker 1: Being "on."

Characterized by: Inability to stop fixing the world, even in your head. You run on the beach on a beautiful day, and your mind instantly starts picking over your friend's divorce, calculating your checking account, planning your next day, and perhaps solving climate change.

Energy effect: Five minutes later, you're drained.

Why we do it: For the "atta girls." In our school days, we got "atta girls" for having our hands up and being front and center. On the job, we got "atta girls" for coming in early, taking on extra tasks, looking perky and bragging about lack of sleep. No surprise Wonder Woman has become our default operating mode, even on the beach. Needless to say, always being "on" comes with a cost. And if we're being real, it's a pretty negative and expensive one.

Weapon of choice: Learning to be present. If you're running on the beach, try locking the world's problems in a mental file cabinet (you can always retrieve them later) and turn to your senses: feel the sand, smell the ocean, taste the salt air, hear the waves, see the sun shine. (You'll learn more about this great mindfulness approach in Chapter 10.)

Blocker 2: What-iffing.

Characterized by: Overuse of two little words: What If. As in, *What if they don't like me? What if I can't pay my mortgage? What if I don't get this fat off?*

Energy effect: See Blocker 1.

Why we do it: Because, weirdly, worry and anxiety are comforting. They make us think we're preparing for the worst, and that surely the worst will happen if we're not "ready" for it.

Weapon of choice: Dismissal. If you'll pardon my language, nine times out of 10, *what ifs* have about as much value as a fart in a stiff breeze. Write down whatever you're what-iffing about right now and put it aside. Look at it in two hours or two months. Chances are whatever consumed you in the moment is gone and forgotten. Or play out the worst-case scenario in all its glory—but then don't forget to add the all-important tag: "Now what?" The truth is, even if the worst happens (*Oh, my God, they hated my presentation!*), guess what. You'll go to sleep, wake up, and try again. This truth was a sobering one for me.

Alternate weapon: My favorite version of the Serenity Prayer: "God grant me the serenity to stop beating myself up for not doing things perfectly, the courage to forgive myself because I'm working on doing better, and the wisdom to know that you already love me just the way I am." It's time to make your faith stronger than your fear. This mindset has been another huge game-changer for many of my clients over the years.

Blocker 3: Holding on.

Characterized by: Overuse of two little words: Used To. As in, *I used to weigh 110 pounds! My husband used to be so romantic! I used to fit in these jeans! I used to have no cellulite!*

Energy effect: Energy wasted tearing oneself down instead of building oneself up. *Instant* drain.

Why we do it: At first blush, saying "used to" sounds like healthy awareness. *I used to fit in these jeans, didn't I? Gosh, I can do it again!* But instead of pumping us up, "used to" soon becomes the soundtrack to our ongoing repeat-dieting pity party.

Weapon of choice: Listening to that wise guy Socrates: "The secret to change is to focus all of your energy not on fighting the old, but on building the new." Ditch the pity party and start accepting you are as you are. You'll instantly gain energy to build new habits and allow old ones to phase out, which is essential for sustaining positive change.

Blocker 4: Perfectionism.

Characterized by: Overuse of three little words: Not Good Enough. Even when people tell you that you look great. Even when you hit that first 10-pound mark. Instead of celebrating your victory, you think, *By God, I'm going to eat like a minnow and get Janet Jackson's 1997 abs!*

Energy effect: A complete waste of it. First, there's no such thing as perfect. Second, in my unscientific opinion, *getting to 99 percent perfect takes about twice as much* *energy as getting to 95 percent.* Think about it. If you want a clean floor, a good sweep would be about 95 percent perfect. But 99 percent perfect would mean lifting every inch of the rug, cramming a toothbrush in every corner, and hunting down every dust bunny like Elmer Fudd on double espresso. Not a good use of energy, I'd say!

Why we do it: Essentially, because we're yo-yo dieters! To us, Photoshopped Celebrity Perfect Body is what "happy" looks like. And having unrealistic expectations of ourselves guarantees that we'll fail and try again. And again. And again.

Weapon of choice: Remembering two things: Perfect is the enemy of good. (Really!) And "done" is better than "perfect."

Blocker 5: Comparing and despairing.

Characterized by: What I call "Terminator Eyes"—the ones that go *beep-beep-beep* when they scan a crowd and land on Miss Snake Hips with her concave stomach and belly ring. Followed, of course, by examining one's own ordinary belly and declaring, "Not Good Enough."

Energy Effect: Don't get me wrong: comparison alone doesn't have to be bad. If someone's running just a little faster than I am, I'm pumped to keep up and see what my body can do. But beware the despair! I had a client whose eyes would swivel at everyone in the gym: *Look at her booty. I'll never have arms like that.* Whenever she did it, I would watch her momentum drain like sand through my fingers.

Why we do it: See Blocker 4, Perfectionism. Plus, we aren't tuned into *our* value and *our* strengths.

Weapon of choice: Reality check, please! I once saw this sign in a feminist restaurant (yes, there were such things in the '80s): ***There are 8 women in the world who are supermodels and 800 million women who are not.***

Furthermore: Be yourself; everyone else is taken. And: Better to be your best than to beat the rest.

Blocker 6: Supporting unsupportive people.

Characterized by: Saying, "Oh, he's just like that," when someone gives you a shot. Or listening and listening (and listening) to someone's drama without noticing your mood dipping lower and lower. Or hanging on to friends who say, "Why do you need to diet? Don't get too skinny, now. Here's a fork for the cheesecake."

Energy effect: Creeping self-doubt, dejection, rationalizing, giving up.

Why we do it: We're just so *nice!* And we hate confrontation, we fear loneliness, we're underconfident, and we don't honor ourselves enough to give toxic "pals" the heave-ho.

Weapon of choice: First, awareness. Notice that drop in mood the next time *that person* texts or calls. Next, action. Stop picking up the phone! As you pay attention to how you feel around someone's energy, it becomes easier to manage your own.

I once had a client who did nothing but complain during my training, particularly about her "cheap" parents (who, by the way, were paying for the sessions!). On the day she said she hoped it would rain during the Oscars so that the celebrities would get "messed up," I borrowed a line from America's favorite sweetheart, Greg Brady, and told her something "suddenly came up" and I got too busy to schedule her. Best career decision *ever!*

Blocker 7: Flaw-seeking.

Characterized by: Fatal self-absorption in the mirror, including pinching one's fluffy bits, poring over perceived blemishes, and contorting one's torso to make one's stomach disappear.

Energy effect: Sets your inner critic off and running. *[Expletive deleted.] I swear, next time I look in the mirror my stomach will be flat, or else. I wonder if I should go a size up in jeans? Would bigger jeans make me look skinnier, or would I be surrendering to the awful truth of my fatness? I wonder what I should have for lunch. Shit, I already had carbs at breakfast . . .*

Why we do it: Because the mirror is right *there.* And it's so familiar to look for the bad, especially after many attempts of trying and failing to lose weight. *And maybe, just maybe this time I'll catch a glimpse of myself and I'll look like Photoshopped Much Younger Celebrity! Wait, I don't?*

Weapon of choice: Pick one: Stop checking in on yourself. (Hah!) Put a post-it on your mirror that says, "I like this person," or "Hello, Gorgeous!" Or have selective, positive vision. Look at your cute nose and beautiful smile. Or call out your body for what it can do instead of what it looks like. Be like my friend who refused to have laser surgery to improve her nearsightedness "because I like not being able to see my wrinkles." Or take a cue from my friend Jill, who looks at her ass as providing "just enough cushion to sit on the bench at my kid's baseball game without hurting."

Here's more from *The Power of Full Engagement*: "The irony is that self-absorption ultimately drains energy and impedes performance. The more preoccupied we are with our own fears and concerns, the less energy we have available to take positive actions." Well said.

Blocker 8: Too much technology.

Characterized by: An hour disappearing every time you go online to just check that *one thing*.

Energy effect: By now, it's an accepted fact that social media is a major trigger of depression. Compare-and-despair, perfectionism, negativity, what-if-worries—it's all there on our friendly phones and laptops.

Why we do it: Because technology beats good intentions. We think *this time* we won't go for the click-bait, we won't check to see College Roommate's perfect life, we won't pay attention to that huge sale at Favorite Online Store, or we won't try to post the perfect selfie with the coolest caption . . . but technology knows human behavior better than we do!

Weapon of choice: Digital dieting. Pay attention when something triggers your self-doubt or lack of hope. For a lot of us, social media can KO our self-esteem quicker than a roundhouse from Jackie Chan. So, notice whether technology is giving you a leg up (great recipes, fitness tips, advice) or a push down (celebrity Instagrams, vacation photos from Fiji).

Bringing the energy back.

Like waaay back. Now that you've equipped yourself against those Energy Blockers, you're just a few steps away from reclaiming *all* your power to stick to your choices and live your best life.

Before we get there, let me give you a short science lesson. Here it is: *Energy begets energy.* Every cell in living organisms contains mitochondria, which convert energy from the sun or oxygen into cellular energy. Without that outside energy, cells cannot grow and reproduce.

By beating back your Energy Blockers, you are, metaphorically speaking, allowing your sun to shine. You're waking up your body and clearing your mind for self-renewal. You are begetting energy!

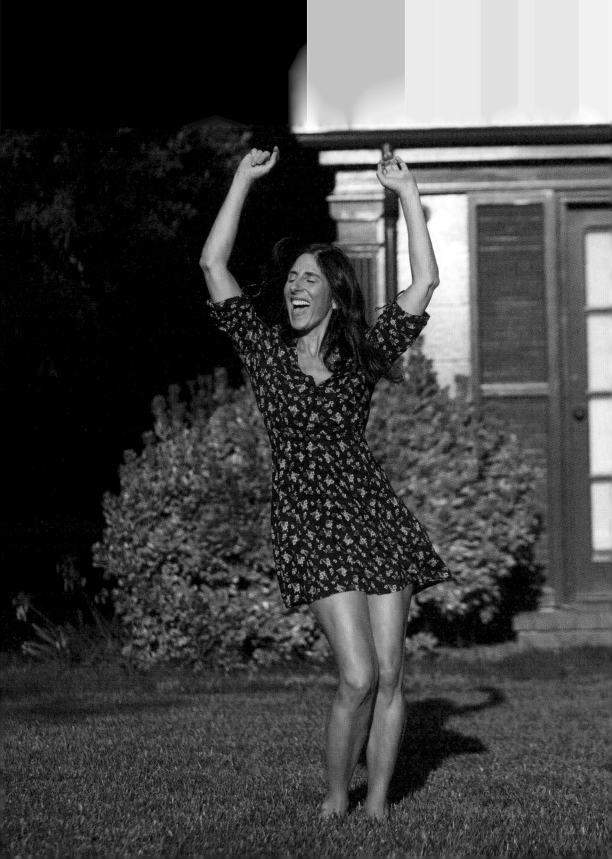

Definition of renewal:

Renewal / noun / re·new·al

1. Replacing or repairing the action of something that is worn out, run down or broken.

Here's where we add in the final steps for self-renewal, self-care, and keeping your energy tank full.

Enjoy!

Self-Renewal Step One: Have fun.

Remember fun? Taking aimless walks, soaking in the tub, playing singles tennis, watching *Sixteen Candles* for the 22nd time? It's all that stuff you used to do before you "realized" you weren't good enough and you "needed" to whip yourself into shape. It's also the stuff you feel guilty doing because you're not producing something or cleaning something or improving something. And yet it's the very stuff you need to renew your energy and create balance in your life.

I'm not here to force you into high-skipping down the street. But I'd like you to start playing with the idea of . . . playing. Because the more positive energy you put into your day, the less you'll want to boo-hoo your way to the drive-thru. This simple little strategy is *the* magic pill solution you've been searching for when it comes to losing weight and living healthy.

Self-Renewal Step Two: Have a feel-good list.

So now let's get some of that fun on the page. Granted, fun may still be a totally unfamiliar concept, especially if your crazy schedule has been running your life. I get it. So for now, all you have to do is write down what makes you feel good.

That's it! And keep in mind: your fun is *your* fun. It doesn't have to be the trendy hiking spot or that movie everyone loves. Your fun is what makes you smile and makes you feel the world is smiling back.

For instance, my friend Kim, a typical Planner, says she hates soaking in the tub. It makes her feel guilty, bored, and *wet.* Her go-to recharger is chopping vegetables while listening to Lionel Richie. My Socializer client Alex prefers to recharge by calling friends while he does an evening unwind walk in the neighborhood. And my client Donna (a Leader) likes to end a stressful day by kicking the shit out of a heavy bag at her boxing class!

And me? Here's my go-to feel-good list:

1) **Running** on the beach. I love being able to push myself harder without the distractions of people and traffic. Running also helps me maintain a healthy weight, which is one of my life priorities.

2) **Watching** *Grease* or *Dirty Dancing*. Guaranteed mood lifter.

3) **'80s playlist**. Dancing. Need I say more?

4) **Playing softball**. Competitive enough for my Leader side and social enough for my Socializer side.

5) **Shopping** at the local farmer's market. Yummy healthy food *and flowers!* I can never have enough yellow roses.

6) **Massage**/day at the spa. Of course.

7) **Walking** Lily, my crazy-adorable boxer.

8) **Binge watching** *Impractical Jokers*. I've seen every episode at least 25 times, and I've totally got a crush on Sal!

9) **Talking** to my BFF Louise. I'm a talker, and she's a great listener.

10) **Jumping rope**. An instant mood shifter and energy booster and goes great with a little Salt-N-Pepa!

Okay, your turn. Write out your own feel-good list, and know this is a judgment-free zone. Think about what might boost you at the start of the day and what might relax you at the end of the day.

Hint: Think like a kid again. When she was eight, my Supporter client Sarah used to love going on the swing set first thing every morning. She's picked that habit up again, on her daughter's swing set, at age 48! Another Socializer, Michele, remembers being comforted by praying the Our Father with her grandmother before bed. Guess what's gone back into her bedtime ritual.

Remember, fun will be the most vital step in creating more balance in your life! When you feel good, you're more likely to carry out all of the goals and intentions you set for yourself.

YOUR GO-TO FEEL-GOOD LIST

1) _____

2) _____

3) _____

4) _____

Self-Renewal Step Three: Schedule it!

Okay, one more thing. Right now, I want you to turn right back to the previous chapter and schedule in your feel-good activities, just as you would schedule a doctor's appointment. And when self-doubt starts to creep in (notice I said *when,* because you're human and it will), ask yourself this: Who do you think is more productive: A marathoner or a sprinter? Marathoners keeping going until they burn out and hit the proverbial wall. Sprinters, on the other hand, maximize short bursts of energy. They renew and repeat. So schedule those short bursts and plan for your success.

1) **When I might do this on a daily/weekly basis:** _____

2) **When I might do this on a daily/weekly basis:** _____

3) **When I might do this on a daily/weekly basis:** _____

4) **When I might do this on a daily/weekly basis:** _____

Self-Renewal Step Four: Express gratitude.

That may sound small, but it's not. We repeat dieters are experts on everything that's wrong, unfair, and awful. After all, isn't that what life has shown us? We've tried and failed and tried and failed to lose weight so many times that we know in our bones that we are inept and the world is terrible.

Except of course that we aren't, and it isn't.

Expressing gratitude is how we check in and know that we are deeply okay. Believe me, that was a very uncomfortable practice at first for this New York girl, taught to detect every kind of rip-off and to believe the worst until shown otherwise. But as I started to treat *myself* better, I noticed things in the world I hadn't seen before. I saw a smile from a stranger. I paid attention when a car let me go ahead. I'd take it in when a client said, "thank you." The more I chose to support my best self, the better the world got.

So gratitude is now a conscious and daily ritual. I prefer to practice gratitude with my morning coffee; it helps energize me to reflect on what I enjoyed yesterday and what I'm already thankful for today. Others prefer a gratitude reflection at the close of the day. But what's great about gratitude is that it's always at hand, and it always works! Even in the middle of a hot, smoggy, Friday rush hour (*especially* at rush hour) I can be grateful for a great song on the radio, the memory of a friend's visit, or that hike I'll be doing tomorrow with my dog. And *that's* the kind of feeling that keeps me from reaching for the ice cream when I get home.

Self-Renewal Step Five: Create a gratitude list

Although you can practice gratitude anywhere and anytime, writing out your blessings is a brilliant way to put them into focus. By putting pen to paper, you're automatically shifting focus from those energy drains (hello, Perfectionism, Flaw Finding, and Not Good Enough) and consciously thinking of the ways in which life has given you love and hope. That's an instant energy booster.

When you make the list, be specific. Of course you can say you're grateful for "my family," but your list is much stronger when you can really see, taste, and feel what you're grateful for. My gratitude list, for example, looks like this:

> I'm grateful for the second chances I've been given in life, or heck, any opportunity I was granted. It's fulfilling to reflect back to all the times I received a "yes" or support.
>
> I'm grateful for the way my dog, Lily, wags her whole body when she sees me.
>
> I'm grateful that the vendor at the farmer's market always remembers which roses I like best.
>
> I'm grateful that my husband always says things that are practical and loving.
>
> I'm grateful for clients who always look me in the eye and thank me.
>
> I'm grateful that yesterday I had ginger tea instead of wine.

Now it's your turn. May your list be long, rich, and ever-growing!

MY GRATITUDE LIST

1) _____
2) _____
3) _____

It's all about balance

A few weeks after you look this over, I'd love you to return to your Energy Pie Chart above. Maybe that self-care slice has gotten a little bit bigger. Maybe you've got more energy for family and healthy living because you've gotten rid of toxic people or relaxed your Terminator vision. Maybe you're even checking the mirror less often! If so, good for you. You're finding balance. You're aware of what's draining your tank, and you're focused more on self-renewal so that you can continue making positive change. So, stick around! The best parts of your journey are still ahead.

The Battery Types: Which are you?

Every personality type has its own way of using and losing energy. Take this quiz and see what fires up *your* batteries.

Your spouse receives an invitation for a 20th class reunion. You:
a) Wonder if you've got a bigger house than everyone else there.
b) Start dress shopping. Fun!
c) Start planning what to do with the kids.
d) Hope you'll have the flu that night.

Your child's teacher asks if you'll bake cupcakes for the Halloween party. You:
a) Tell your spouse to find some nice "homemade" ones at the grocery store.
b) Invite other moms over to decorate them.
c) Make enough to supply the other kid parties you've been asked to bake for.
d) Spend an hour scrolling through recipes to find the exact best one.

You need to schedule plane reservations for a vacation. You:
a) Ask an agent to get you something that leaves at 9:00 a.m. and arrives at noon and no stops, please.
b) Start chatting up the reservations person. Has she ever been to the Grand Canyon?
c) Won't use that *other* airline, even though it's cheaper. You need to *know* the airline you're using!
d) Go into Travelocity heaven (for you) and after two hours emerge with a $120 fare. Okay, it's five stops and two airlines, but *look at the savings!*

You have to hand in a report in the morning. You:
a) Will put someone right on it.
b) Bitch and moan and pull your hair out. Those Excel spreadsheets—who can figure those out? Besides, *you're missing the neighbor's barbeque!*
c) Do an excellent job, as usual. Been there, done that, know how it goes.
d) Will have to ask for an extension. You found some very interesting tangential information that needs to be followed up.

You've been asked to be a maid of honor, or best man. You:

a) Treat the situation as if you're CEO of Wedding Inc. Everyone has a role, people, so get to work!

b) Are super-duper excited. Parties! Dresses! Shoes! All eyes on me! I mean, the bride . . .

c) Will fit all that *work* in, I suppose, and don't you think my little Susie would be a nice flower girl?

d) Are completely flummoxed. Where's the instruction manual on how to do this correctly? I don't want any mistakes!

If you've checked mostly A's, you are indeed Ms. Leader. You're the alpha dog who gets energy from taking charge. If you preferred B's, you're the Socializer, the one who gets energy from others. Those answering with C's are Supporters, the ones who get drained when life takes them off their routine. And the ones who checked D's are Planners and think happiness is the details.

Now that you know your energy type, take a look below to see what will keep you in peak form, ready for positive change!

. . . .

BATTERY TYPE A: THE LEADER

Energized by: Action. Decisiveness. Delegating. Big-picture thinking. Competition.

Drained by: Details. Indecisiveness. Unfinished projects. People who can't get their point across. To-do-list minutiae. Anything *small*.

Tips for peak energy:

1) Delegate the small stuff, or at least break up the tasks so that you're not doing one after another. A call to the cable company followed by standing in line at the Post Office will wipe you out quicker than a 5K run.

2) Schedule phone/Internet time and stick to it. Constant checking for updates that don't push you forward robs you of your excellent focus.

3) Take a break. Period. Leading, directing, controlling, organizing—stop being a slave to achievement. Off time is just as fruitful and valuable as building the Guggenheim.

BATTERY TYPE B: THE SOCIALIZER

Energized by: Friendships. Admiration. Parties. Impulsive fun.

Drained by: Routine. Schedules. Big, amorphous tasks, like report writing.

Tips for peak energy:

1) Stick with your peeps. Exercise with friends, eat healthy stuff with friends, shop for workout clothes with friends. Make your healthy lifestyle a party!
2) Cut down on "yes." You're always being asked to chair this committee or plan that party. And yes, you'd *love* to do it all. But you can't. Put yourself first.
3) Steer your impulses. When you go shopping, all hell breaks loose. So shop the farmer's market, maybe, instead of the MegaGoodiesMart. Bring friends for support!

. . . .

BATTERY TYPE C: THE SUPPORTER

Energized by: Knowing what to expect. Favorite routines. Family and close friends. The dog. Doing what you're good at.

Drained by: Abstract, big-picture tasks. Unknowns. Tackling unfamiliar projects or unfamiliar situations.

Tips for peak energy:

1) Schedule for balance. Make sure you include your self-care in your to-do list and schedule your workout for the time you're least likely to be asked to drive someone to the mall.
2) Keep the refrigerator stocked with easy, healthy choices. Don't reward yourself for "getting everything done" by ordering in pizza.
3) Learn "no." You spend the day making sure everyone's got everything they need. You've earned that long walk—and okay, take the dog if it makes you feel less guilty.
4) Stretch just a little. Try a new recipe, a new type of workout, even a new restaurant for the family. The break-in routine will be energizing, I promise!

BATTERY TYPE D: THE PLANNER

Energized by: Detailed, purposeful tasks. Curiosity. Problem solving. Control.

Drained by: Impulsive behavior. Abstract problems. Unpredictability.

Tips for peak energy:

1) Make yourself into a learning project! Research nutrition and exercise, then choose programs and recipes and *track the results*. There's a wealth of material to explore, and you'll enjoy it.

2) Remember: "Done" is better than "perfect." Striving for perfection—in that report, that project, that task—eats up valuable energy. Try going for 95 percent and then move on.

3) Relax your expectations. At some point, the cable guy will need to come back, *again*. At some point, someone will scratch the car, *sometime*. At some point, some waiter isn't going to remember you asked for water. Life happens. Roll with it. Save your energy for things you enjoy, like managing QuickBooks.

. . . .

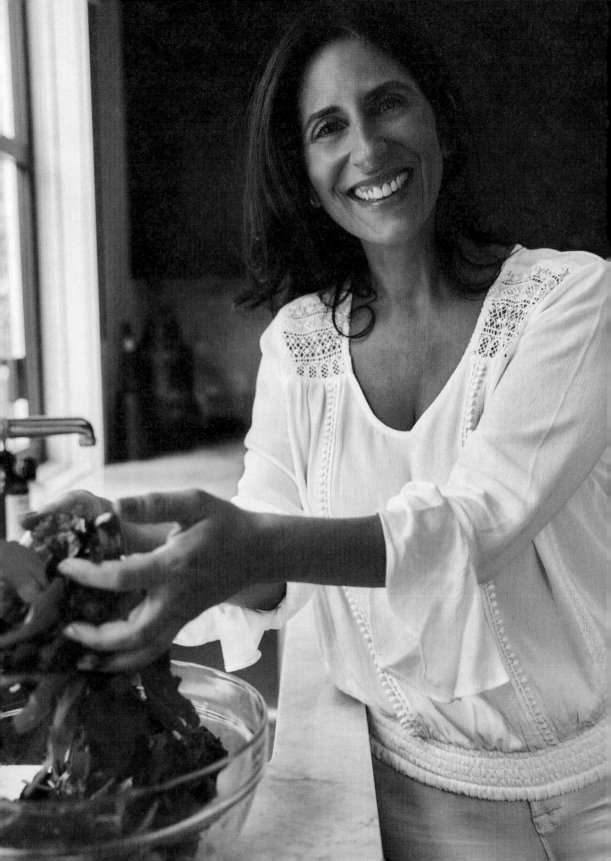

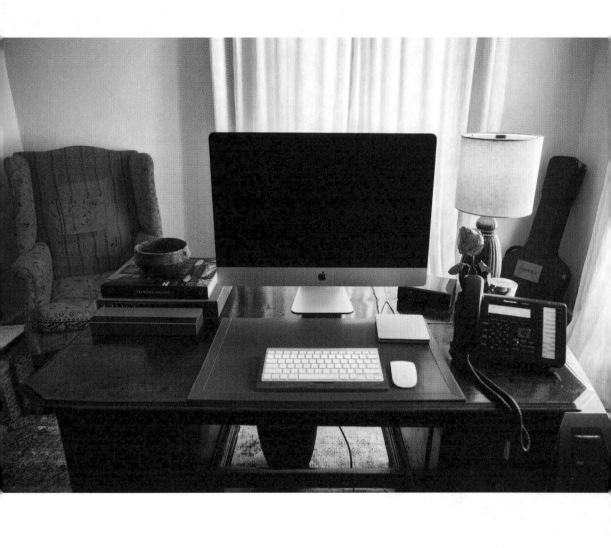

CHAPTER SEVEN

When You Get Clean, You Get Lean—For Real!

■■■

The Bigger the Waste, the Bigger the Waist!

OKAY, I'M SURE THERE ARE energetic, productive, lean, and healthy people out there who live in complete chaos. In fact, I know one excellent fitness trainer who has probably not seen her car upholstery in years, thanks to the accumulation of kettle bells and yoga mats.

But believe me, those people are exceptions. *Clutter drains energy.* It's as simple as that. You say you don't believe me–you behind the stack of unopened mail, months-old magazines, and piles of charger cords? Let me ask you a question. Do you not sit a little straighter behind the wheel right after you've vacuumed your car? Do you not breathe relief from your shitty day when you see your cleaning lady has paid a visit? And do you not then feel a little bit more badass, a little more in control of your day and life?

Many of my clients come to me in a state of lingering overwhelm. There was Kelly, who said she just could not understand why she had no energy, no time, and an extra 20 pounds that stuck to her like a lamprey eel. She was young, she was healthy, she was smart–what the hell was wrong? So I paid her a visit at home. After I parted the sea of chip bags and soda cans (no surprise there), I saw bags of fabric and a dusty sewing machine. I saw stacks of unread books and papers. I saw dishes piled on counters and recycling piled on the floor. I even saw a pair of jeans in an open closet that I *knew* hadn't fit her since the last millennium. And in the middle of it stood Kelly, looking hopeless. No wonder! It was as if every object were screaming, "Deal with me already, you loser!"

Here's the thing: clean is transformative. It really is! A chaotic space is a nag and a drag, a constant reminder of everything we're bad at and dislike about ourselves. That project we'll never get to. That invitation we forgot to answer. That $250 jacket the salesperson talked us into that we wore once. The Facebook "friends" from fifth grade. Who needs them? Even talking about it is exhausting.

But a clean space lightens you. It gives you permission to focus on your best self, instead of that pile of crap. When you have a tidy space, an organized schedule, a leaned-out pantry, and a closet of flattering clothes (instead of those mocking size 2 jeans), you are ready for real change. That's why, when I visit a new client, one of my first instincts is to grab a broom. (Sweeping is also a calorie burner, which I'll get to later.) We play some music and have fun, but make no mistake: This is an act of revolution! This is a freedom rally against all the old stuff and old habits that weigh us down. Literally!

And that's what happened with Kelly. As we cleared up her house and life, she stopped trudging and moaning. Her mood lifted and she moved with a new lightness. It was as if—*bing!*—a spark of possibility had entered her life. Adios, suffocating piles of stuff. Hello, energy! Her weight loss journey began that day, with every dish we put away and every chip bag we tossed.

So this chapter is about controlling *your* overwhelm. It's about freeing up the precious real estate in your head and life that's been taken over by stacks of laundry, unread emails, and endless kerfuffles over homework and who walks the dog. It's also about freeing you from the more insidious energy blockers in your life, like the board games you and your husband *used to* play, the bike you thought would change your life, or the hideous vase your aunt forced on you. I'm 100 percent serious when I say this stuff is making you unhealthy. In fact, it's making you *fat*. It screams, *You suck, you never finish what you start, and you and your husband need therapy*. It gives you yet another reason why you end up dialing Domino's instead of heading for the gym.

And by the way, that's not just theory: in his book, *Lose the Clutter, Lose the Weight*, expert organizer Peter Walsh writes, "I find the problem is that homes are littered with broken promises and way too much stuff. It causes us to feel sad and stressed, and the link between those emotions and being overweight is now a scientific given." The good news: when you clear away the stuff that doesn't serve you, you make room for what you value and cherish—namely, YOU!

Let's grab that theoretical broom and get going.

Step One: Know the Enemy!

Essentially, clutter assumes four guises in your life:

1) The physical *things* around your house, car, garage, what-have-you.

2) The unhealthy *foods* around your kitchen.

3) The energy *blockers* around your workspace.

4) The time-suck *relationships* that creep over your boundaries.

What's lousy about clutter is that it spreads. If you have it in one area of your life, you almost certainly have it in another. Ever notice, for instance, how you can never leave messages with the office manager who can't find his stapler beneath the landfill on his desk? Or how your friend with the Where's Waldo garage always has lost souls camping out on her couch?

But that's also the great thing about clutter. When you start clearing out one area of your life, the other areas begin to take care of themselves. The assistant who dumps her desk-top landfill, for instance, is the one who'll remember what you like for lunch and whether your package is due today or tomorrow. Guaranteed!

So let's take a look at what clutter is doing in *your* life.

The Clutter of Things

Nobody is born naturally tidy (except perhaps freakishly neat Marie Kondo, author of *The Life-Changing Magic of Tidying Up*), but everybody has a different way of coping with physical chaos. Let's look at some of the main players in the vicious Circle of Clutter (as identified by Walsh) and see if any of these have taken up residence in your home.

Lazy clutter: also known as, the stuff you'll get to "later."

Examples: Unopened mail, clothes in the dryer, that spatula that lives in the dishwasher because there's no room left in the drawer.

Often found in the home of: The Socializer. She's so busy driving field trips and planning girls' nights that—good grief, where did all those bills come from, anyway?

Coping strategy: Get in the tackle-it habit. Try the Take Five method from household-advice guru Heloise. Either set a timer for five minutes and clean up what you can (and hey, if you go longer, that's fine), or just do five things in your line of sight. Easy-peasy!

Memory clutter: also known as, the stuff you "can't" get rid of because it was from Grandma/Aunt Dinah/my kid/our vacation.

Examples: The ugly crocheted potholder, a chipped Tiffany bowl, a purple crocodile from art camp, a math test with an A-minus.

Often found in the home of: The Supporter. She's all about family, so tossing out Baby Susie's onesie (she's 14) would be like forgetting she was ever a baby!

Also found in the home of: The Planner. She's so good at organizing bills and papers, but what are you supposed to *do* with that sweater Granny made, or that shoebox full of menus from when you and hubby were dating?

Coping strategy: Okay, Supporters: keep in mind that *things* are not *memories*. I had one Supporter pal who actually kept her grandmother's *phone*—yes, the kind you plug in—after Grandma died. As it turned out, my friend was still able to remember Grandma just fine after sending the phone off to recycling. And she gained counter space for a vase of Grandma's favorite flowers!

My Planners, meanwhile, ought to put those excellent organizing skills to work on compiling albums and sorting through piles. Buy some boxes and dedicate one nice, long, methodical session (or two) to going over the stuff. Call in another organized pal if you need back-up!

I-Might-Need-It-One-Day Clutter:

Examples: A Pack 'n Play, 10 yards of gingham curtain material, a waffle iron, six extra duvet covers.

Often found in the home of: The Leader. Frankly, a Leader doesn't usually get that attached to memory stuff, but she does wonder if maybe those squash racquets will make it back to her workout. She also points out that the decorator *did* pick out that fabric, the waffle iron came in handy once, and hey, that ski rack cost $700! You can't just throw that stuff away!

Coping strategy: Get practical. Go through the house, put all the "someday" stuff in a pile, and sort out what to donate to charity, what to sell at a garage sale, or what really makes sense to keep on hand. If you really love that curtain fabric, call a tailor *today*. You'll feel in control again, and control is what motivates you Leader types to stay the course with positive change.

Malignant clutter: also known as, the stuff that reminds you of breakups, illnesses, or other painful times.

Examples: High-school diaries, pictures of you and Bad Boyfriend, a signed cast, the coaster from the restaurant where you broke up.

Often found in the home of: The loyal Supporter. Supporters often feel that reminders from the past can put them in control of it.

Coping strategy: Ditch it! Remind yourself that your malignant clutter is not in line with your core values or who you are today. When you let go of yesterday's negative energy, you choose to engage differently and more healthily today.

Clean House Workout

You say you can't get to the gym? *And* your dust bunnies have joined ranks with last month's pretzel mix under the bed? Boy, are you in luck. As I once demonstrated on the *Today Show,* household chores like sweeping, vacuuming, and folding laundry can become a full-body workout. For real! Check these numbers, which represent calories burned per 30 minutes:

1) **Washing floors:** 187 calories.

2) **Scrubbing the tub:** 180 calories.

3) **Vacuuming:** 119 calories. Burn more by lunging and adding wrist and ankle weights.

4) **Sweeping:** 184 calories.

5) **Cleaning windows:** 167 calories. Plus, who doesn't *love* clean windows?

6) **Wall washing/painting:** 167 calories.

In other words, a solid hour of housework burns about as many calories as a half-hour run. And you'll kick that evil clutter to the curb!

Bonus Core Workout: Folding Laundry. Sit on the floor with the laundry basket on one side of you. Lean back, engage your abs, twist toward the basket, fold the item, then twist to your folded pile on other side. You get three types of crunches *and* folded clothes. For added challenge, lift your legs or lean back farther. Contract your abdomen, engage your pelvic floor, keep your back straight, and remember to breathe!

The Clutter of Food

Yes, food *can* be a clutter problem. And if you don't believe me, I challenge you to open any cabinet—go ahead, I'll wait—and see if any of these items are inside:

* Something expired.

* Something you don't remember buying.

* Something you planned to eat but never did.

* Something with more than five ingredients in it.

* Something with more than two multisyllabic ingredients.

Yep, that's clutter. And no matter what else you may find to argue about, I think you'll have to agree that it's a pretty straight line between a leaned-out pantry and a leaned-out physique.

So here are my kitchen rules for leaner and cleaner:

The refrigerator is king.

It's where most of your food should live. Why? Because if your food is shelf-stable, it's processed, and if it's processed, it's not the best choice. *You know this.* Healthier food choices have five or fewer ingredients, and true whole foods have just one ingredient and need refrigeration in order to keep.

Skip the smell test.

If it's past its expiration date, toss it!

If you can't pronounce it, denounce it!

Beware the following ingredients: monosodium glutamate (MSG), trans fats, high-fructose corn syrup (HFCS), sorbitol, aspartame, saccharine, sucralose (Splenda), and sugar alcohols like erythritol. If Great Grandma didn't cook with it, don't eat it!

Divide and conquer.

Personally, I hate seeing more food than I can eat. What person ever consumes two whole celery hearts? Food piles and mystery containers mean hassle, and hassle means forget it, I'll just eat leftover pizza. So when you buy food, divide it! Portion it out into containers or freezer bags. Then you can grab what you want when you want it. No prep, no fuss, no feeling that you lost control of your food plan. And I love my glass containers: they're BPA free, you can see what's in them, and they make colorful veggies look as good as dessert. Well, almost.

Become a spice girl.

Spice is what lets you become a foodie *and* fit. I am not kidding when I say I prefer a hard-boiled egg with smoked salt to a bacon-and-cheese omelet. And don't forget the fresh stuff, like cilantro and basil. Check out recipes online or at the back of this book, and when you see a spice or seasoning you've never heard of, go for it.

When you're prepping for positive change, these rules matter! In the end, your cleaner, leaner pantry will mean you'll see a whole lot less waste. And yes, you'll see less of your *waist* as well. (I know. I went there.)

The Clutter of Work

I think we can all agree: work is stressful. But your work*place* doesn't have to be. With my clients, I see an inverse relationship between messiness and efficiency: the cleaner the space, the more work gets done. Plus, the more efficient they are, the more fit they are! Efficient people have time and energy for self-care, *and* they have the satisfaction of accomplishment. That's a one-two punch for living your best life.

To be at your best, then, you need to set the stage for a great day. Here's what I suggest:

* **Downsize your to-do list.** Make it no more than five items per day and prioritize what *must* be done and what *should* be done. Long lists guarantee failure and frustration. Short ones ensure success.

* **Create a positive "eye space."** Clear the clutter from your line of vision. Add in flowers or an inspirational quote or photo. Just remember: one or two photos are fine; 20 photos make you cross-eyed. (Ever notice that the fancier the store, the fewer the number of items in the window? It's how retailers say, "Attention: This is important.")

* **Corral your email time.** Pick a time of day that you'll tackle that message pile and stick to it. Send an automated response explaining that you'll be in touch later. One client removed her work email from her phone, and another refused to listen to phoned-in complaints and demands. She uses Voice to Text instead so she can scan the messages stress-free.

* **No more pings and dings!** Get rid of the apps that take you out of the moment. Ditch the dings, bells, and notifications. Are you more efficient now than before you knew about Instagram? I thought so.

* **Change the meaning of "crunch time."** True fact: the longer the computer session, the stronger the urge to crunch. This is prime Doritos time. Stave it off by having something healthy-crunchy on hand: baby carrots, kale chips, cucumbers, home-popped popcorn. You *will* become full and control the mindless binge-fest!

* **Learn to cry "Uncle!"** Respect yourself enough to know when you need a break. Say no to driving carpool three extra days. Say, "Sorry, can't," when the boss moves the deadline. Let someone else take the class gerbil home. And guess what: the world won't end if you play hooky for a day! In fact, you'll perform better if you're well rested and clear.

The Clutter of Relationships

I'm sure you're a nice person. How do I know? Because nice people attract energy-sucking people the way a statue attracts pigeons. See if any of these scenarios sound familiar:

* *Your neighbor always parks in front of your house.* (You: "Oh, it's fine.")
* *Your mom friend never picks up her kid on time.* (You: "She's so busy.")
* *Your coworker regales you daily with boyfriend drama.* (You: "She needs a friend.")
* *Your old buddy from high school just can't get it together!* (You: "She tries.")

Here's what's true about each of these people: *Not one of them puts you first.* They aren't supporting you, they aren't cheering you on, and they're siphoning the resources you need to live your own best life. These relationships are toxic clutter, pure and simple.

Remember, "You First" is what this journey is all about. You simply can't have a healthier, fitter life if you're giving your precious time and energy to people who don't give it back. You can't!

Now that you're living cleaner and leaner, you need people who support you and want to see you at your best. To weed the energy suckers from the energy boosters, try this simple method adapted from *The Life-Changing Magic of Tidying Up*. Author Marie Kondo suggests decluttering your space by taking each of your objects in hand and asking, "Does this spark joy?" If the answer is no, out it goes!

Now, "Does this spark joy?" is pretty clear when you're opening a jar of Nutella, wearing your Like A Virgin tour T-shirt, or sitting on the 405 Freeway on Friday afternoon. So I say we apply the question to our relationships, as well. Close your eyes, bring that "friend's" face into view, and ask yourself:

* *Does this friendship enhance my life in any way, help me achieve my goals, or make me feel supported?*
* *Does hanging out with this person spark joy?*

Better yet, try these variations:

* *Does it spark joy when I'm working overtime on my boss's project while he is yachting?*
* *Do I need a Xanax just to look at my coworker's face?*
* *Does this smirking salesperson really care about my footwear needs?*

* *Does this so-called boyfriend make me want to binge every time I am near him?*
* *Have I ever belly-laughed with that Eeyore?*
* *Would I rather stick a fork in my eye than have this person on my team?*

I think you get the picture.

Your path to positive change should look like the last mile of the LA Marathon. You want everyone on it pumping fists, yelling, *You rock!* and *You're almost there! and You got this!* What a difference it makes when you surround yourself with people who have your back, who aren't jealous when you lose weight, who make you smile just thinking about them, who are on your team.

I know it's easier said than done. It took me four decades to figure out who is on Team Christine. But to start clearing out your relationship clutter, just remember, you deserve joy. We all do. So trust me when I tell you that the cleaner your life gets, the leaner you get.

Stay tuned, because I've got more joy-sparking tips on the way.

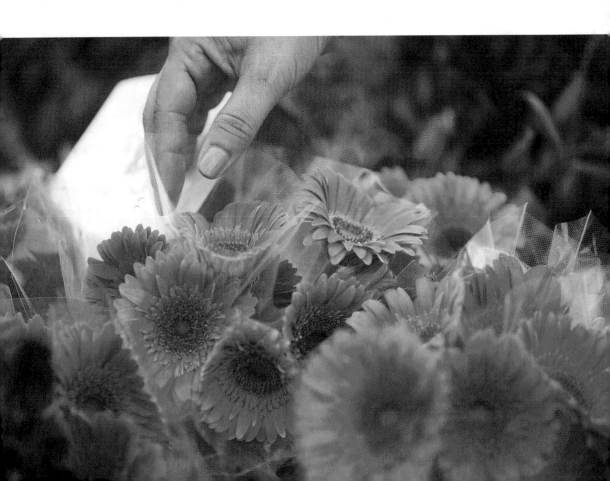

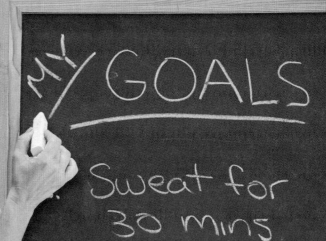

MY GOALS

1. Sweat for 30 mins

2. 5 Mins of Gratitude

3. Sign up for Singing Lessons

CHAPTER EIGHT

Your Goals: Make Them, Rock Them (and Okay, Revise Them)

■ ■ ■

Say It with Me: Fantasies Are Not Goals!

LIKE MOST YO-YO DIETERS, I used to give myself an A-plus in goal setting. I mean, wasn't I setting goals *all the time?* Lose 15 pounds. Gain a six-pack. Run 10 miles. Get Cindy Crawford's body. (Yes, that was a goal once upon a time. It was the '90s. Don't judge.) Of course I failed at all those goals, but I sure was great at making them!

At the time, these goals made perfect sense to me. I was always the "chunky" one in my pretty friend group, and even in my family. My sister was so skinny she had to wear long johns to fill out her jeans. My mother has never weighed an ounce over 118. Of course my body should be exactly the same as theirs, right? I must not be trying hard enough!

Naturally, I didn't know (or didn't believe) that I had a completely different body type. So I didn't have "goals" at all; I had fantasies. What business did I have trying to look like Cindy Crawford? I mean, I'm five-foot-three. I grew up putting butter on my steak and eating candy as if it were the last food on earth. And most important, I'm me. Why did I not accept that, no matter how many crunches I did, my musculature will never form a six-pack? I had to learn the hard way that if my goals weren't in line with my personality, priorities, and lifestyle—not to mention my genetics—then they weren't goals at all. They were just setups for failure, and failure was something I thought I completely mastered.

Over the years, I've also learned that goals are not "shoulds." If I tell myself, "My goal is to have a flat belly," what I'm really saying is "If I don't have a flat belly, I am a loooooser." A true goal is one that feels good and makes sense to *me* and me alone. It's something that I want to achieve for helping myself live my best life.

It can be challenging to sort out goals from "shoulds." For instance, when was the last time you made a goal that didn't involve comparing yourself to, say, Miss Flatbelly in your yoga class? Or the last time you made a goal that wasn't based on a perceived outcome, such as "If I lose this weight, my Bad Boyfriend won't leave me?"

These days, I make sure that all my goals align with a single idea: becoming my best self. That may sound simplistic, but the truth is that most repeat dieters pursue goals that work *against* themselves. They're trying to get skinny because someone told them they should. They're slogging away at the treadmill, trying to emulate some Photoshopped celebrity. Or they're trying to get skilled at something trendy, like boxing or bodybuilding, that they hate doing or isn't natural to them. Remember, this whole journey is about you, with your own unique values and personality. A true A-plus goal is one that will feel good to you the moment you start going for it.

One more thing: when your goal feels right, it's a lot easier to get to the finish line! Your mindset switches from "have to" (*I have to hit the treadmill—God, I feel like a hamster trapped on a wheel*) to "like to" (*I'm loving this kickboxing class! I feel like Superwoman!*).

So in this chapter, I'm going to show you the SMARTER way to goal setting (yes, that is an acronym!). No more wishes and fantasies. No more setting yourself up for failure. Now that you've assessed your own values, habits, and priorities in the previous chapters, you're ready to move the dial in ways that increase your confidence and keep you pointed toward your own best self.

SMARTER goals are better goals

Originally used for establishing business objectives, SMART is a well-known system that stands for Specific, Measurable, Attainable, Relevant, and Time-bound. The idea is that a SMART goal—one that hits all the buttons—is an achievable goal. And with that in mind, I've created the SMARTER (like you!) goal-setting system. It's my belief that SMART goals should *also* be Energizing (so that you're really pumped about working on them) and Revisable (so that you can build in needed flexibility).

Here's how SMARTER breaks down.

SPECIFIC. A vague goal is no goal at all. "Cutting down on bread" or "walking more" are not exactly the flags that will rally the troops. Your goal has to be worded so that you can say, "Yes! I did that!" Whether it's "lose seven pounds" or "run a 10K" or "compete in a Spartan race," your goal needs to have a *there* there. Think about exactly what you want to achieve. Define it. Revise it. Then see yourself doing it. When you can state something solid and specific about what you want to accomplish, you have yourself a goal.

MEASURABLE. Here's where your goal starts to take on real dimension. If you want to run a 10K, what pace do you want to hit? If you want to lose seven pounds, how many calories will you need to cut back? By giving yourself parameters—"I want to run a Spartan Race in under two hours"—you're ensuring that you're really in the race, and that a celebration victory lies ahead.

ATTAINABLE. This is a good one. The unattainable goal—looking like Cindy Crawford, perhaps?—is *the* reason repeat dieters end up back on the couch with a bag of Cheetos. Goals have to be realistic enough to be achievable, but challenging enough so that victory is sweet. So, if you're 40 pounds overweight, don't give yourself the goal of losing every pound in three months. Start with an achievable, celebrate-able goal of, say, 10 pounds in two months. Make it a stretch, but keep it real.

RELEVANT. This step helps clarify whether this goal really matters to you and you alone. If you want to run a 10K, for instance, ask yourself why. Is it because you're naturally drawn to running and enjoy competition? Or is it because your friend is running the race and talked you into it? As you set your goals, keep your values and priorities first and foremost. If your goal is not a natural fit, or if you're doing it to please someone else, you might want to choose a different goal.

TIME-BOUND. Like a race, every goal needs a starting line and a finish line. If you're starting today on your goal, when's the finish? Will you lose those seven pounds by next month, or in three months? Will you hit a nine-minute mile in six weeks or six months? Ask a pro for input at this stage—a coach, trainer, or nutritionist. You need a time frame that's both realistic and challenging so that you can set a pace for victory.

ENERGIZING. Let's face it: all of us would love to just snap our fingers to drop 10 pounds. Wouldn't any of us rather eat a brownie than a bell pepper? But here's the thing: meeting a goal is waaaay more satisfying than a brownie binge, particularly if that goal is one you want to achieve *just for you.* So make sure your goal is one that you're really jazzed about. (Don't care about running? Skip the 10K and set another goal!) And keep setting minigoals within your goals, and celebrate. If you go without donuts for a week, treat yourself to a mani-pedi at the *nice* salon. Remember, you're in this for the long haul, so make every day a victory for *you.*

REVISABLE. Goals need to be victory tapes, not brick walls. If your new job means you can't hit the gym four times a week, you might need to push back that time frame on losing 10 pounds. If your honey surprises you with a Bermuda cruise, that November Spartan race might be out the window. But even when life happens, hang onto your goals! Flexibility is not copping out. Flexibility is *working with.* It turns a set*back* into a set*up.* The gym is still there and the stationary bike is missing you. When you hit a snag, reset, revise, then recharge. Your goal can handle it!

A WORD ON FLEXIBILITY. You've heard me say it before, and it's worth repeating. For any positive change, you need a flexible mindset. This is a growth mindset, one that allows for positive action, increased confidence, and the ability to know when you've had too much and it's time to play. It lets you meet yourself where you are *today.* So if today the ghost of Julia Child offers you a slice of a homemade baguette, with butter made from Belgian cows eating Irish grass, I suggest you drop your no-carbs resolution. Go ahead. You have my permission. We need this BFF relationship with ourselves because every day is different, and what matters is *consistency,* not rigidity. Being emotionally flexible is the most worthwhile tip I can ever provide you. It's the true difference between success and repeated failure.

Let's get to work!

Whatever goal you choose, your first exercise will be the following: Pick up a pencil. You're going to write down exactly what you plan to achieve, how, why, and when.

Why write? It's the best way to keep yourself accountable. If your goal is *no candy for two weeks,* seeing it in black and white keeps it from morphing into *no candy with red wrappers* or *no candy containing xanthan gum.* Also, writing your goals increases your chances of reaching them. Ever notice that your itemized to-do list always gets done? And it's so satisfying to cross those tasks off one by one.

So let's get started creating and refining your SMARTER goal. Remember, this is for the long term, so I'll guide you through to make sure it's a perfect fit for your values, lifestyle, and personality.

Step One: Name a specific goal!

It doesn't have to be perfect at this stage, but it does have to be strong, specific, and long term. Let's say you want to drop two dress sizes. Can you visualize what your body will look like at that size? Can you see yourself in the clothing you'll wear? Do you see yourself moving and living in that body size?

Now write your own goal: _____

Step Two: Take measurements.

What kind of calorie count might you need to reach this goal? How many hours per week would you need to exercise? Think hard about which steps might be involved in reaching this goal. You can't reach the finish line by ambling all over the track, so be specific about what you're going for. Then, as you take off, continue to keep up the momentum by measuring and monitoring your progress.

Specify the measurements to achieve in this goal: _____

Step Three: Make sure it's attainable.

Are you really ready to drop two dress sizes? Think about what's involved: gym time, shopping lists, saying no to cheesecake. If it feels overwhelming or discouraging, or if it's just a bad time to start planning extra workouts, think about revising your goal to something that's in easier reach. No pressure!

How does this goal differ from previous goals that you didn't achieve?

_____

Why do you think you can reach this particular goal?

_____

Do you have the time, space, equipment, and mindset to reach this goal? If not, what do you need to do to make it happen?

_____

Step Four: Make sure it's relevant.

Spend a moment thinking about why you want to drop two dress sizes. Is it because your spouse thought you looked heavy? Or is it because you're tired of carrying around extra weight and you're not comfortable moving around in your body? Make sure this goal resonates with you and you alone.

Why does this particular goal feel right? How does it differ emotionally from previous goals that you didn't achieve? Review Chapter 3 for ideas on identifying your core values.

_____

Step Five: What is the time frame for this goal?

Now that you know specifically what steps are involved, how soon do you think you can reach your goal? Make sure you account for holidays, vacations, work schedules, and other potential distractions. And check in with your trainer or coach! You might think you can drop those sizes in two months, but your coach has the experience to know what you're really capable of.

Specify a realistic time frame for this goal. _____

Step Six: Are you enthused?

This is an easy one. Is this goal something you're dreading, or something that pumps you up? If the idea of achieving this goal makes you feel excited, then you're good to go!

What excites you about achieving this goal?

_____

How might you keep yourself motivated if you start losing that enthusiasm? (Hint: Make it a priority!)

_____

Step Seven: Is your goal revisable?

Emotionally and physically, it pays to be flexible in reaching your goal. Try to anticipate which habits or events might throw you off track. Then assess your progress and results as you go. Should you revise your expectations? Do you have a Plan B in mind just in case you can't fit in all those workouts? Are you willing to give yourself more time to drop those dress sizes, or would that feel like a failure?

What events or situations might cause you to need to revise this goal?

_____

In case I get thrown off, my Plan B goal is:

_____

BREAKING IT DOWN

Some people approach their goals the way Michelangelo carved marble. They chip away day after day, week after week, no results in sight, trusting the process. When they're done, *voilà!* They look and feel magnificent.

Most *normal people*, however, approach their goals the way Chain Saw Chucky carves a bear out of a log. They're not working too hard and they're not getting anything great out of it, but at least they're trying! Sort of.

In short, most of us have no patience for reaching goals. Instead of going all the way toward a David-like outcome—say, a 25-pound weight loss in three months—we'll settle for the chain-saw bear equivalent of a couple of pounds.

But actually, it's not that hard to get back to Michelangelo mode. The key is breaking down the goals. Instead of going to the three-month finish line all at once, ask yourself: What can I achieve in the next month? Or the next week? Or even the next day?

My client Tina, for instance, had a goal to run three miles in 25 minutes within three months. Her current pace was 37 minutes, so we made it a goal to get to 35 minutes by the end of the following week. We then cut the time minute by minute every other week until she met her 25-minute goal. One minute doesn't seem like a whole lot over three miles, but in the end, she cut her time by 35 percent!

Minigoals have three important functions.

1) *They keep you on pace for reaching the brass ring.* You won't drop 25 pounds in six months if you're still up 20 pounds at five months. You need that minigoal of dropping five pounds in one month, and then another five the month after that.

2) *They indicate whether your goal is attainable and realistic.* If Tina couldn't hit a 10-minute mile after three weeks of hard work, she probably would have needed to dial back her long-term goal. (Goals must be revisable, after all!)

3) *They give you more opportunities to celebrate!* Every minigoal achieved is another reason to give yourself a pat on the back and a special treat. (Even if it's just looking in the mirror and saying, "You rock!" because you passed on the pastry, or worked up a sweat for 30 minutes!)

So take your goal and break it down. Ask yourself:

What's my long-term goal and time frame? _____

What do I want to achieve today? _____

What do I want to achieve next week? _____

What do I want to achieve next month? _____

My reward for meeting each of those goals: _____

_____

Then, go for it!

Goals, intentions, and YOU

Whether your goal is to drop a dress size, ace your math final, or buy a house, you must start with *intentions*. If a goal is a destination, intentions are the path. They are the attitudes and behaviors that get you to your own personal pot of gold.

Let's say you want to save for a house. Before you start figuring out how big and how much (goal setting), you need to have an *intention* of thrift (or, conversely, of earning). You need to get comfortable with the idea of budget making, or of taking on a part-time job. Those intentions will then help you buckle down and start putting money aside.

Same with weight loss. Before you pick a specific size or number, you're going want to create intentions that are specific to you *and* your goals *and* what you value. Such as:

I intend to put food in my body that is healthy.

I intend to stop eating when I'm 80 percent full.

I intend to break a sweat at least three times a week.

I intend to schedule "me" time 20 minutes a day.

I intend _____

Notice that these intentions don't have a finish line. They're your signposts that will keep you on track to your goal and will continue to serve and support you even after you've dropped that weight. They represent your true long-term plan to respect and achieve your best self. And they give you flexibility! Because intentions are not hard and fast, you have the choice to take them or leave them as the day unfolds.

This freedom *really* helped me out of my yo-yo nosedive. Previously, I'd made my goals so rigid (Ms. Perfectionist, after all) that I would dread getting out of bed to face them. (*Please, God, make the treadmill disappear!*) Now I use my intentions to "play" toward my goals, rather than death-march to them. I make every choice on how I feel *now*. When I get to the workout, I set a goal just for that session. Wow—what a difference that makes for black-and-white thinkers like me.

Here's another way to think of it: Intentions bring focus to your process and performance. Goals focus on the outcome.

But of course, different personalities are going to take different approaches to goals and intentions. So, if the goal is, say, to lose 10 pounds, here's what that might look like:

For **LEADERS**, that 10-pound goal will be waving in front of them like a toreador's red cape. (Picture Dr. Phil here, head lowered, pawing the ground.) Forget squishy intentions; Leaders are all about action. But once they learn that, nope, they can't delegate someone else to run on the treadmill, Leaders will find that they'll need to lean on their intentions for support.

So if you're a Leader type, make sure you're clear about what you're doing and why you're doing it. Don't kick yourself because you didn't hit your 10-pound mark on the first try. Once you really accept that your intention is to live a healthy life, you'll charge right back at your goal again.

SOCIALIZERS, my warm and nurturing friends, will cozy right up to intentions. Of course, they'll have an enthusiastic attitude about treating themselves with healthy love. (Picture Oprah here, toasting her goals with her gal pals.) The only itty-bitty problem, however, is that action is a little challenging for these social types, particularly when friends invite them for desserts and wine.

So if you're a Socializer, you might want to enlist those friends to put a little accountability into your program. Make sure they know and support your goal. Intentions are great, but only behavior will kick those 10 pounds off.

The **SUPPORTERS** need routine in order to reach their goals. More than other personality types, the trick for them is to create healthy habits. (Picture your favorite soccer mom with a carload of balls, dirty uniforms, and bags of cheese sticks.) Once they've adopted an intention of eating lighter and moving more, they need to make sure the refrigerator is stocked and the workout time is blocked out.

If you're a Supporter, then, beware of your old habits coaxing you back. Shift your behavior bit by bit toward your intention of staying active and healthy. Like your Leader pals, you need inner motivation for support, and outer structure to keep you on track.

PLANNER types are all about structure, too. In fact, they're happiest when they have the steps outlined and the progress journal open and ready. (Here's your estate lawyer, pencils sharpened, white-out bottle close at hand.) But follow-through—well, that can be tricky for these Planner types. Before they really get going on their goals, Planners practically want a signed guarantee of success.

So if you're a Planner, double down on your faith in the process. Decide exactly *how* you're going to exercise and eat better (e.g., "I will spend half my grocery budget on nonprocessed food") and keep track of your progress. Don't worry if the pounds don't fall off immediately; as long as you stick to your intentions, your goal is there waiting for you!

Final note: Of course, we're all hybrids when it comes to goals and intentions, but I'm betting that some of these tips resonated with your own unique values. So keep that pencil in hand and write your own intentions. Think of it as your personal mission statement not only for reaching your goal, but for living your best life. Acknowledge who you are and where you would like to be. Be gentle, be real, be enthusiastic!

CREATING A VISION BOARD

To see something is to want something. Every retailer knows this. Funny how we don't "want" any shoes until we see that glorious set of heels in the store window, or how we weren't even *thinking* about pastries until that French éclair came into view!

Fortunately, we can also stimulate our eyeballs—and our impulses—for our better selves, as well. With a Vision Board, you get your desire working *for* your best self, instead of against it. And you get to choose the message.

So grab some cardboard, scissors, and magazines (or Pinterest photos) and create, ideally, three different Vision Boards. I have just two rules:

1) *Stay positive.* In other words, if you want to be more active, don't put up a picture of a couch with a big "X" through it. Your subconscious will register the couch, not the "X." Use a picture of someone running, dancing, or moving with energy.

2) *Keep the body images real.* No six-packs. No skinny-mini 18-year-olds. No *Sports Illustrated* swimsuit models. I don't even want to see Christie Brinkley, who in her 60s is still a freak of nature. All of that leads straight to the Land of Compare and Despair.

Now, to work!

Board Number One: A *daily inspiration* board of goals and intentions. Show healthy yummy fruits and vegetables, flowers, your family. Show images from your favorite hobbies (paintbrushes, yarn, bikes). Put anything up there that keeps your daily frame of mind upbeat and confident of achieving what you love.

Board Number Two: A *no-holds-barred* fantasy of what you would love in your life. I don't care if it's horses and castles, mountain streams, a marathon medal, and a pet elephant. When you're finished, look for patterns and ideas that line up with your values and priorities. See if they connect with any goals, potential or current. (Perhaps a Swiss hike and side trip to Africa?)

Board Number Three: A *goal-setting* vision of yourself. On this board, you'll put on images of what you'd like to accomplish during the next six months. Maybe, if you want an acting gig, it's a vision of you on TV. If you want weight loss, it's a vision of the clothes you'll want to buy in the size you're gunning for. If you want to run that Spartan race, have a picture of the medal. Finish the board, and six months later congratulate yourself!

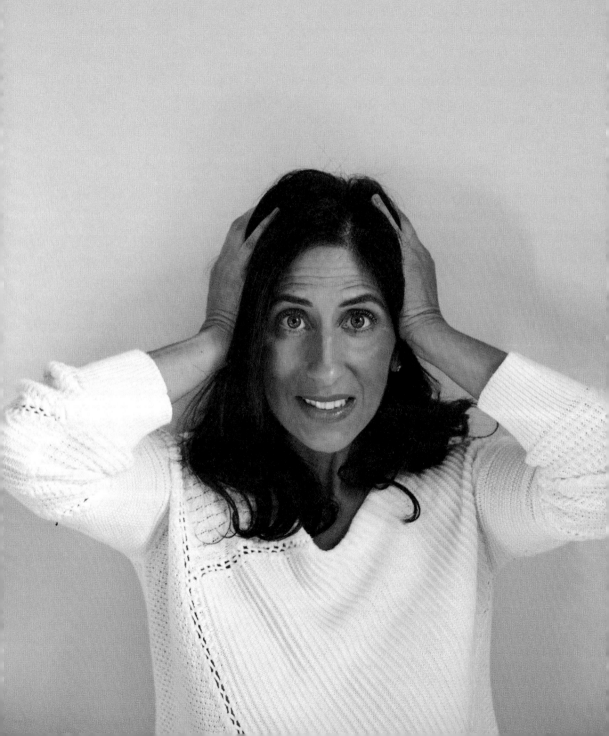

CHAPTER NINE

Dear Voice in My Head: Can You Shut the F*** Up!

■■■

Stay Out of Your Head: It's a Bad Neighborhood!

YOU KNOW THE DRILL. New diet, new workout plan—*hey, world, look at the new me!* (Cue theme to *Rocky*.) *I can't wait to hit that treadmill! Bagels be gone! I crave watercress and chamomile tea. Carrots, yes!!*

And then . . . *Boy, that treadmill is a grind. Hmmm, there's leftover lasagna and birthday cake in the fridge. (Rocky theme scratches out.) Oh, man. I'm so out of shape. This is the worst time to start a diet; the holidays are coming up, and there's so much traffic on that road to the gym. I've never lost this stupid weight, and I never will. I've been at this since I was 13! When does it end? I'm such a loser . . .*

This, my friends, is not "you" talking. This is your inner bully, always ready to stick out her foot and trip you right off your best intentions. Psychologist David Burns calls it Stinkin' Thinkin'. Writer Anne Lamott calls it Radio KFKD (yes, that means K-Fucked). It's that personalized channel in your head that blasts a constant stream of all the things that are wrong, shameful, and awful about you, you, you.

And it's not just your channel. Every yo-yo dieter is tuned to KFKD day and night. *Fine. Eat that ice cream. You'll never get a flat stomach anyway. I can't believe you. Get a life!* It's not only the voice of defeat, it's the voice of "why even try?" It convinces you that you just can't do it, so you might as well go finish off that leftover birthday cake.

But yes, there is good news. The truth is, once you start hearing your self-talk, you can heal it. Just as you weed out the energy drainers and the time wasters, you create inner peace by weeding out the image bashers.

This is critical for positive change. Think of it this way. Which kid is more likely to win a swim race: The one who hears, "Oh my God, what is the matter with you? You call that kicking? You should have stayed home, you loser"? Or the one who hears, "Okay, just a little further! You can do it! Focus—you're almost there!"

Let's face it: Negative thoughts lead to negative actions—or in some cases, negative non-actions, which keep us from our goals. And if you're aiming to get healthy, you've got to think healthy to make it a reality.

So here's how.

Step one: Get to Know Your KFKD classics!

Stinkin' Thinkin'—cognitive distortion, in psych talk—is universal. Each of us has a brain that is excellent at coming up with ways to make us feel unworthy, pessimistic, and defeated. But yes, we can shake it off like T-Swift once we learn to recognize the lingo. Do any of these KFKD classics ring a bell?

It's All or Nothing

Sounds like: Whoa, girl, you scarfed down that cake! I don't care if it's your birthday: this is spinach-and-quinoa time! You'll have to run 90 minutes on the treadmill tomorrow. You're going to blow everything.

Variation: You did only 15 minutes on the elliptical instead of a half hour? It doesn't count. Damn it, you'll have to do 90 tomorrow.

Why it's a KFKD classic: It turns tiny lapses into black-and-white catastrophes. Catastrophes create stress. Stress makes it likely you'll relapse. And then you're either "on" or "off" your diet in a heartbeat. Which leads to a pity party for one, with pizza.

Change the channel to: My personal favorite tune: "Flexibility." If you did only 15 minutes of working out today, kick in another five minutes tomorrow. If you had a piece of cake, no big deal. A blip in the routine is just that, a blip, not a reason to declare defeat and raise the white flag. Just pick up where you left off. It's not the cake that throws you off; it's the rigid thinking.

Shoulda, Coulda, Woulda

Sounds like: Wow, running is harder than I thought. Look at those girls cruising down the sidewalk—I should be like them! Why am I so bad at this? I could've been a faster runner if my parents had encouraged me to stay on the track team!

Variation: Oh, I would have had a kale salad for lunch, but everyone else was having a burger.

Why it's a KFKD classic: It creates false expectations and unrealistic demands. Which leave you feeling defeated and unworthy. Which leads to another pity party for one—this time with ice cream and cake!

Change the channel to: Getting real. Expectations are disappointments waiting to happen, and the higher the expectation, the harder you kick yourself for "failing." Look at what feels good and makes sense for your age, lifestyle, and body type. Trust yourself to do what's best for you, not what's best for someone else. And if you made a choice you regret, decide you'll do differently, and move on! Every moment, every day, brings another opportunity for a new choice.

One more thing: My fave swap for *should* is *preferable*. As in: *It would have been preferable if I chose to eat the kale salad instead of the burger.* This quick reframing takes out the condemnation and gives you the freedom to switch it up next time.

It's All My (or Their) Fault

Sounds like: Hey, I didn't pick the all-you-can-eat buffet! She did! And what am I supposed to do? If I'm paying for chili and ribs, I might as well eat them!

Variation: If my boss weren't so horrible right now, I would really get right on that new diet plan. But I'm too stressed to add more stress to my life!

And: If my kids didn't have baseball practice, soccer practice and dance, I'd have time for myself.

Why it's a KFKD classic: It lets others dictate the terms of your life, health, and choices. Then you can blame them when you "fail." And finally, you can feast on your anger, resentment, and shame at another all-you-can-eat pity party.

Change the channel to: Putting on your big-girl undies. Take responsibility for choosing what's in your best interest, not theirs. Your life. Your choice. You can do this!

It's Too Late to Change

Sounds like: I have never been able to do more than five push-ups. There's no way I'll lose this 10 pounds. I mean, I'm 50! That's just what happens at this age.

Variation: Really? You expect me to eat kale? It's too late for this extra-Caesar-dressing lady!

Why it's a KFKD classic: It creates a fear that new habits will make things worse instead of better. Or it assumes you are incapable of change, which means you might as well just give up the dumb idea of working out and go have a pity party for one, with more pizza and extra pepperoni.

Change the channel to: Trusting. Yes, you are aging, and you can respect that—but you can also choose how age will look on you. All humans have the capacity to change. And as you've been learning throughout the book, change comes a lot easier when your efforts and goals are in line with what is meaningful to you. New choices just might energize you, inspire you, and change the way you look and feel about yourself. Dare to go there.

I'm a Lame-o

Sounds like: God, you're sooooo [favorite insult].

Variation: Oh, why did I [favorite lapse]? Woe is me.

Why it's a KFKD classic: This label-making spin is more intense than the teacup ride at Disneyland. It assumes we are dull and powerless in a world otherwise populated by shining stars. It leads to feelings of defeat, regret, "there you go again," or "I suck." Sigh. Bring out the violins and cue the pity party, this time with margaritas!

Change the channel to: "Oh, well. So you ate those cookies. At least you learned that it's a trigger for you when your mother calls. Next time, have some carrot sticks nearby." Your awareness is a catalyst for making new choices.

It Wasn't Good Enough

Sounds like: I only swam five laps. That girl was still in the pool after 10.

Variation: I swam five laps. Next week, I must do 11!

Why it's a KFKD classic: It's the perfectionist's BFF. it creates unrealistic expectations and a false assumption that your efforts aren't ever good enough. Which means you "fail." And you get a permanent pass on the I'll-Be-Happy-When Roller Coaster. *And* you win a seat at a pity party for one (add your vice here).

Change the channel to: Reality. Someone out there will always achieve more than you. Someone will always achieve less. Who cares? Maybe Extra Laps Girl just polished off an entire wedding cake. All that matters are *your* goals, feelings, and intentions. Set the bar where it's a stretch for you, not for Diana Nyad.

Overgeneralization

Sounds like: I'll always be lazy/fat/unmotivated/etc., etc.

Variation: I'll never be able to fit in a workout/stick to a diet/find time to meditate, etc.

Why it's a KFKD classic: It concludes failure and tells you to give up before you even start. How could you possibly predict you will always fail? Do you have a new job as a fortune-teller? Life becomes an unending pity party, this time with pizza, drinks, cake, and a pack of smokes.

Change the channel to: Anything with a "maybe" instead of "always" or "never." As in, "Maybe I can fit in a workout." Or, "Maybe I can go without that second glass of wine." When you say "maybe," you at least give yourself possibility and hope.

Time to Change That Tune

Radio KFKD isn't the only culprit when it comes to our lousy self-image. Some (seemingly) innocent everyday words carry their own little poison darts. These trigger words can drop us faster than Ronda Rousey against Holly Holm. See if they crop up in your own self-talk:

Skinny/fat. Clearly, one implies the other. If someone's skinny, that's indicates someone else (like the person using the word, perhaps?) is fat. Who wants that?

Say instead: Ideally, nothing. They're both judgments about what a person "should" weigh. Every time you say, "I want to be skinny," you're really saying something is wrong with you. Nothing in life is either/or, and that includes you. If you want to build yourself up, avoid words that tear you down.

Good/bad. Again, one implies the other, and to the benefit of neither. Besides, to say "gluten is bad" (unless you have celiac disease) or "Paleo is good" is essentially meaningless without context.

Say instead: "Helps/doesn't help." "Serves me/doesn't serve me." "Works for me/doesn't work for me." "What I prefer/What I don't prefer." Keep the judgment out of your self-talk and save it for the courtroom!

Success/failure. These are particularly unhelpful when they imply all-or-nothing outcomes. "Success" does not mean you've been tapped by the Finger of God and are a superior being. It only means that you've accomplished a particular goal. And "failure" doesn't mean you're destined for life with a shopping cart full of recyclables. In fact, it doesn't mean anything at all: not reaching your goal only means that you're still working on creating the best outcomes for yourself. If you're trying, you're never failing.

Say instead: "Awesome, I did it! I accomplished what I set out to do! I rock!" And, "Well, I didn't make it this time, but I'm still in it to win it. Plus I've learned a lot about what works and doesn't work for me." See the difference?

Must/Should/Would/Could. These "musts" and "shoulds" lead to anxiety, depression, shame, guilt, low self-esteem, self-pity, you name it.

Say instead: "Prefer," "preferable," or "ideally." This eliminates the assumption that things were supposed to go perfectly and completely according to plan. Instead of assigning blame for something going wrong (which "should" implies), you're reframing. Now it's a situation that you'd "prefer" ended up differently. Now it's not your responsibility, it's just your opinion.

. . . And it was horrible/awful/the worst. When "confessing" to a misstep, almost every repeat dieter loves to add a brutal tag, just to hammer home how horrible and awful they are. For example: *I ate cake, and it's a terrible thing.* Or: *I had to walk my last mile, and it sucked.* We treat each little slip like it's a missile launch from North Korea.

Say instead: These two words: *So what?* No need to call in the National Guard just because you did only 10 minutes on the rowing machine. What's done is done! Step back, observe, and tell yourself you'll make a different choice next time. Move on!

Any stupid, random thought about yourself that you believe. Huffington Post recently stated that the average person has 50,000–70,000 thoughts per day. What HuffPo doesn't say is how many of those thoughts are worth a speck of dog poo on the bottom of your shoe. Yet so many times, our thoughts steal our self-worth the way a school bully steals our lunch money. Worse, we then spend our hard-won energy and effort trying to make friends with the bully! We start believing and trying to change our thoughts, not recognizing them for the fictions they are. If you tell yourself, "I'm a strawberry," are you really a strawberry? Certainly not, but that's as big a fiction as saying, "I'm a loser because I ate a piece of cake." Come on.

Say instead: You are not your thoughts. That brain spin is just the result of neurons firing. When you can observe your thoughts with detachment (see the next chapter), you can decide what's worth hanging onto and let the rest float away. Also, when your thoughts get really judge-y, ask yourself: What's the evidence? This cognitive strategy has been transformative for so many repeat dieters, including me!

In short, put some flexibility in your self-talk. And create a new classic station called I [Heart] Me! When you hear yourself saying, "I blew it," or "I look awful," or "I have no willpower," catch yourself, give yourself a little apology, and try a different tack. Say, "I'd like to do a better job next time." Or, "I would have preferred to work out, but didn't get the chance" Or, "My three-mile walk today was just as good as my run."

Trust me, this simple shift in language has been one of the most effective strategies I've used, personally and professionally, over the past 15 years. This bait-and-switch gives you permission and freedom to move forward without getting stuck in a negativity trap. Treating yourself with kind respect (I mean, would you ever tell a good friend, "Boy, you look horrible?") is the first step to living your best life.

Accentuate the Positive

Quick quiz: Which of the following statements from your last job review are you going to remember:

1) Great job on the Millman report.
2) You're showing some real people skills.
3) Your presentations need a little refining.
4) You had some good ideas at the last meeting.

Yes, I thought so. "A little refining" might as well be in red neon. We are all heat-seeking missiles when it comes to negatives, and we toss positives right out the window. Studies show that in marriage, you need five positive interactions—a back rub, an unexpected hug, an "I love you"—to counteract one "Honey, is that cellulite?"

Rest assured: Positive statements do work. But much of the time, we have to work at taking them in. Unlike negatives, which sail into our brains without any assistance, positives need coaxing and a firm place to land. We have to really hear and believe positive statements—whether we hear them from ourselves or from others—before they can help us make positive change.

Here are some ideas for flipping the switch.

Reframe the negative. I always used to see repeat dieting as my biggest weakness. I was ashamed of how often I'd tried and "failed." But guess what. Now I know it actually shows resilience. I know without a doubt that I do not give up when it comes to positive change! And that's a piece of self-talk I can take to the weight loss bank.

Believe the compliments. I know your Socializer friends toss off niceties the way babies toss Cheerios, but guess what. That doesn't make those niceties less true. And when you hear a "You look great!" all you have to say is "Thanks!" You don't need to buy the person a drink, admire her shoes (unless you want to), or say, "Oh, my hair is awful! How can you say that?" You just have to take it in. And practice letting it feel good! You're worth it.

Look for the good. Sure, we're expert flaw seekers, and you know what? Our info-filled world doesn't help. (Ever pick up a newspaper and say, "Wow! Check out all the good news today!") So this may be hard, but trust me, it works: Try to look for the good in every situation. If your dog peed on the floor, treasure the kiss she gave you. If your kid threw up on your bed, remember how beautiful he looked sleeping there. Train your brain to hold onto goodness.

> *Our experiences are all we will genuinely remember*
> *for years to come. Why not make them worth the memory?*

Give yourself a pat on the back. When you're doing your gratitude practice (see Chapter 7), make sure you put yourself on the list. Recognize your worth. Own your contributions. Tell yourself you're a heck of a good egg. Trust me: The more often you feed your own soul, the more positivity and optimism will shine out of you. I want you to be singing Mariah Carey's "Emotions" as you strut down the street.

And conversely, minimize whatever went wrong in the past. There's a reason your windshield is much larger than your rear-view mirror! Acknowledge your mistakes, but keep moving forward, and trust that your positive mindset will carry you along.

Stay emotionally flexible. In other words, don't decide ahead of time how you're going to feel about anything, whether it's your workout, your hair, or your lunch date. When you say, "Oh, I have to run three miles," or "Oh, I have to enjoy this party," you're denying your emotional reality. If you don't really enjoy the party, or you don't really feel like a three-mile run, you'll probably beat yourself up for "failing."

A healthier strategy is to simply meet yourself where you are. If you need to walk after one mile of running, walk! Nobody's keeping score (except your inner critic, who needs to step off). If your yoga instructor keeps picking apart your pigeon pose, find another class! Respect your feelings, celebrate what you can do, and free yourself from judgment. This flexibility has been my single best strategy, personally and professionally, for making consistent progress. As I like to tell clients, "I want to see a short-term memory and big-picture goals."

Choose kindness over pleasure. Out-and-out negatives are easy to identify. Calling yourself a worthless idiot, for example, has zero upside. But what about, say, drinking a milkshake? It sure feels good going down, but those after-effects—self-doubt, shame, guilt, self-pity—are pretty painful.

So next time you're about to take action, ask yourself if what you're about to do is pleasurable or kind. If it's merely pleasurable, it probably comes at a cost. (Which is why I say, "When in doubt, go without.") But if you're choosing an action that's kind to yourself, like a long walk or a massage, then go for it. Put yourself first, not your appetites. (You'll find more ways to tune into your "I [Heart] Me" radio station in Chapter 10.)

Visualize it! Positive self-talk is great; positive self-imagery is better. That's why sports psychologists for years have helped athletes visualize hitting that ball, sinking that putt, making that ski run. The idea works: if you can see it in your mind, you can make it happen in your life.

So, don't be shy! Get out those inspirational photos and put them on the wall. Tape a post-it with "Hello, Beautiful!" on the bathroom mirror. Put your Vision Board (see Chapter 8) front and center, with all those wonderful goals on display. Meditate and "see" yourself moving and eating with pleasure.

And in the end, remember this: We've worked years to perfect our negative self-talk. No one is more expert at pushing our own buttons than we are. Positive self-talk and imagery won't turn that around overnight, but it will keep those fingers off the buttons! So start today, and know that every loving message you give yourself will take root and help lead you off the diet merry-go-round forever.

ROLL THE HIGHLIGHT REEL!

When I met my client Monica, she needed a morale booster, STAT. For half her life, she'd been trying to lose 100 pounds. Her KFKD classics were blasting louder than a Bon Jovi reunion concert. So we created a Highlight Reel! We wrote down every one of her positive attributes: her kind nature, her resolve, her beautiful smile, and her willingness to work hard, not to mention her physical strength. Then we made sure she reviewed it every day to remind herself that she was worth the effort of positive change.

Highlight reels are turbo thrusters for positive self-talk. When you really focus on what you (gasp) like about yourself, you quit giving the lead role to your Mean Girl voices. You tell yourself, "Yes, I'm really worth that extra coaching session. Check me out!"

Of course, if you've had KFKD on each of your preset buttons, creating a Highlight Reel may seem a challenge. When you're used to beating yourself up, the only "highlight" you might be able to muster is "good driver." If that's the case, try these tips:

1) Enlist friends. They'll be happy to tell you what's great about you. Write it down and believe it!

2) Reframe negatives. Almost all traits have a positive side to them. Try these:

   Spontaneous instead of *impulsive*

   Steady instead of *risk-averse*

   Forthright instead of *loud* or *bossy*

   Thoughtful instead of *introverted*

   Thorough instead of *perfectionistic*

   Creative instead of *scattered*

I believe all traits are worthwhile. We're all diamonds in the rough, and from time to time we just need a little polishing!

3) Keep the list just for you. No one's grading you, no one's comparing you. Don't go around checking if your highlights are better or worse than someone else's.

Here's my Top 5 Highlight Reel. This took a while.

1) I am resilient
2) I am loyal
3) I am hardworking
4) I am a fast runner
5) I am a great friend

Now it's your turn.

1) I am _____
2) I am _____
3) I am _____
4) I am _____
5) I am _____

The next time you hear one of your KFKD classics, or you go down the rabbit hole of comparing your behind-the-scenes work with someone else's highlight reel, take this out and consider it the playlist to your new I [Heart] Me station!

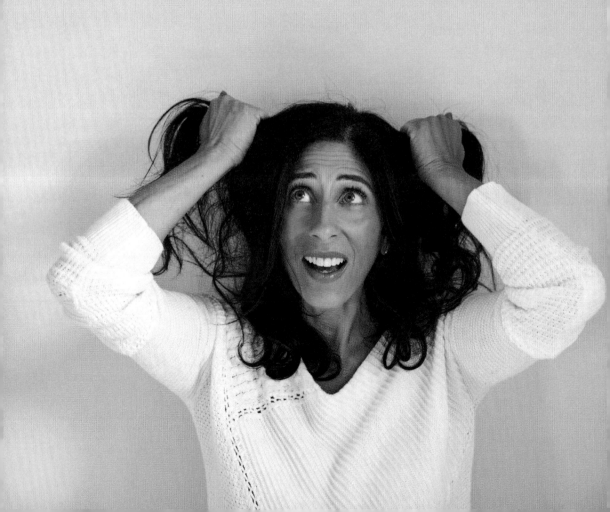

CHAPTER TEN

Calming Your Kinda Crazy

■■■

Stress Relief without Milkshakes: Yes, It's Possible!

Situation: Your bipolar boss sweeps into the office, accusing you of being the schmuckiest assistant since George Costanza. *Oh please, not again,* you think as she unloads both barrels onto whatever's left of your self-esteem. *FML!*

Response: Five minutes and six demands later, she slithers out like the serpent she is; you make tracks to the vending machine.

Situation: Driving home from 11 innings of kid pitch, *waaay* past your kids' bedtime, you hit a red light that is longer than menopause. Perfect time for your little one to bite the older one on his throwing arm, and then it's full-on WWE in the back seat. You fanaticize hitting the pedal to Mach speed and drop-rolling yourself out of the moving car, but *lucky you* . . . saved by the green!

Response: At home, quiet and alone at last, you hunt down your kids' five-month-old Halloween candy, chase Swedish Fish with a shot of Cuervo, and set the alarm for 5:30 a.m. to finish a report. You're living the dream!

Situation: Grab hold of that soaked worm! Your mother-in-law calls to tell you she and her two sisters, Mary and Mildred, will be arriving for the weekend, and oh dear, didn't your hubby tell you? Mary's hip is at it again, so don't forget she'll need to sleep in your bed, but that's okay, right, dear, because even though it's obvious you've put on some weight, you can still fit into the twin bed with the baby (who is 10!).

Response: You blast Rage Against the Machine and drive to McDonalds in lieu of breaking down completely and buying a pack of smokes.

I don't know about you, but my blood pressure shot up just reading that. *Stress!!* And just in case you missed it, I'd like to point out a connection here—actually, more of a welded-steel bond—between *Stress* and *Really Bad Choices.* In my many years of coaching, I've come to believe that the inability to manage stress is the No. 1 cause of all diet failure. No . . . correction: it's the cause of *all* failure. No one has ever had a bingefest because they were having a great day. Our emotions are so complex and difficult to contain in any given moment that we look for outward coping mechanisms—food, alcohol, online poker, marathon Zappos sessions—to help swallow them down.

Of course, stress is a given. You're going to have lousy days at work, spousal arguments, soccer practices, traffic delays. What's *not* a given is your response. Do you *really* need Kahlua milkshakes to cope with a rotten day? No! The intent of this chapter is to help you learn to talk yourself off the ledge and drop the Doritos. They're not here to help!

I know, I know: At a tough moment, a deep breath will never be as satisfying as a Thin Mint. But whatever your stress, whatever your personality, there *is* an effective strategy to help you keep calm and nutrition on. You'll learn to observe your emotions, not act them out or drown them in onion dip. You'll begin to turn your impulsive and irrational *reactions* into mindful and practical *responses* that help you keep your path to achieving your best self. Basically, you'll learn to lighten up when stress gets really heavy.

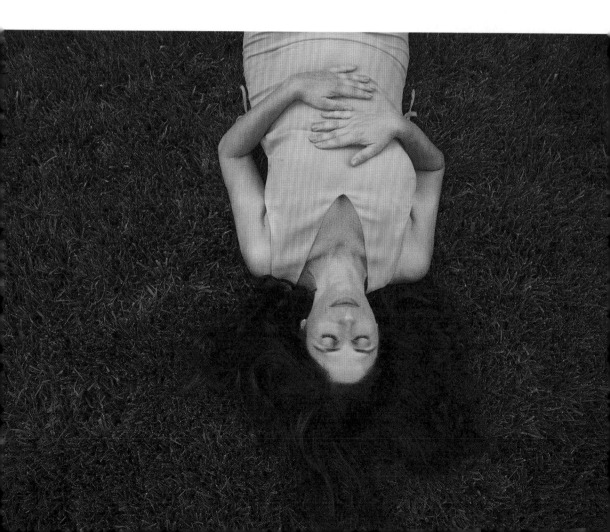

Turn reaction into resilience

Every stressful situation is basically a two-parter. The first part is the stressor itself: The idiot who doesn't understand turn signals, the snow day with three bored kids, the boss who thinks Mother's Day is the perfect time to send you to Duluth. The second part is your *reaction*. And if your KFKD station is on preset, that snow day and business trip are going to send you straight to the cookie aisle. Why? Because you're going to hear "Baby, You're No Good," "Help," "I'm a Loser," and all those other classics that typically accompany your favorite, fully catered pity party.

Granted, you now have some tools for dealing with Stinkin' Thinkin' (see Chapter 9). You've learned some strategies for turning down the volume, and maybe, once or twice, you've even picked up a few static-free minutes of I [Heart] Me. However: When you're dealing with hard-core stress, you need more than strategies: You need resilience. And by resilience I mean *the ability to bounce without making a federal case out of your feelings*.

For wisdom on this, I like to turn to that master of self-compassion, Mister Rogers. (Yes, him.) "There's no 'should not' when it comes to having feelings," Fred Rogers poignantly wrote. "They're part of who we are and their origins are beyond our control. When we can believe that, we may find it easier to make constructive choices about what to do with those feelings." In other words, Mister Rogers is telling us that we all have the ability to be mindful of our feelings: to stop, take note, identify, accept, and move on. We don't have to bathe our anxiety in Frappuccinos or swallow our anger with extra pepperoni. When we're *mindful* about our stress and feelings, we're no longer at the mercy of them.

So slip out of your Keds, get into your comfy cardigan, and know that what's ahead is a beautiful day in the neighborhood.

Zen and the Art of Mindfulness

Before I began my own mindfulness quest, my only encounter with Buddhism had been ordering fried rice (five cartoon chili peppers, please) from the Buddha's Delight take-out menu. My disconnect is precisely why I interpreted the Zen Buddhist concept of "living in the moment" as "living *from* the moment." Every day was spent worrying, speculating, and fantasizing about what I should be doing five years *from now,* five pounds *from now,* five jobs *from now.* Instead of living in a Zen state, I was living in an I'll-Be-Happy-When state. Picture it. I lost my first 10 pounds and barely noticed it, so I changed my goal to 20. *Bam.* Time for a new goal! I ran five days a week, why not six?

Happiness was never where I *was*—it was always out there and out of reach. You can relate, right? So many of us get caught up in the "from now" disease. When we live that way, it's like we're prisoners of our own making, scraping tally marks into concrete walls, counting down to the "day" we will be [better, prettier, fitter, richer] from now. Which is only true if you are Rob Lowe.

When I truly began studying the Zen principle of mindfulness, I finally got it. Happiness was living *in* the now. Of course it's great to prepare for the future: we all need hope, a stocked pantry, and a savings account. But when dealing with stress, we need to dial out of the idea that I'll Be Happy When. We need to sit with where we are and find peace and happiness within. That's what creates resiliency.

And if that's too woo-woo for you, consider that mindfulness does have tons of scientific backing from academics worldwide, from UMass Medical School to Oxford. Their research strongly suggests that mindfulness reduces current stress reactions while cumulatively building our resilience—that inner strength necessary to keep our future stressors at bay.

If I Can Do It, So Can You!

Believe me, I came to mindfulness the hard way. My old-fashioned New York Italian family, while loving, was not exactly long on empathy and compassion. Hysteria was my family's default mode: if someone couldn't find the garlic or lost their keys, it was like Blame of Thrones around the house. And if you felt like you were going crazy at any point, you didn't say you were going to talk it out in therapy, and you didn't dare bare your feelings. You made your own wine or punched a wall. *What's the problem?*

Needless to say, I stunk at self-regulation and had no inner resources to control my stress. By 21, I was experiencing panic attacks and mild agoraphobia. You know how you ring that ding-y thing on the bus to get off? Well, I rang it, except I was on the Bronx River Parkway at the time. *Ding Ding Ding. Get me off this goddamn bus. I can't breathe! I can't go to work!* I cried so hard that day because I was stuck, both on the bus and in my imprisoned mind. I did see a therapist, and while I certainly valued the suggestion of medication, I sought more. I really wanted to find a way *out* of that place in my head where my Inner Wall-Puncher kept telling me I was no good at getting through life.

I'm happy to report that mindfulness really moved me past those growing pains. In fact, it helped not only with my mind, but with my body, my food, and my fitness. Having a detached awareness of my feelings, thoughts, and body sensations gave me the ability to dip my toe into places that felt uncomfortable at first, like exercise. I could listen in to my cravings and know whether they were about physical hunger or emotional neediness. I felt, for the first time, as if I could really understand and care for the real Christine.

Mindfulness practice, as woo-woo as I thought it was at first, was the key to getting me out of my prison. And if it worked for this girl, it's going to work for you!

And here's why.

Mindfulness lets you tame the beast within. If you can name it, then you can tame it! By bringing awareness to your thoughts, mindfulness lets you step back and identify what exactly you are feeling: "I feel resentful that my boss takes me for granted." That simple action gives you the detachment to *see* your resentment without taking it so literally and *without* hitting the vending machine. (Thich Nhat Hanh talks about this concept in his book *Taming the Tiger Within*.)

Mindfulness helps you stay in tune with your body. Stress causes emotional distress, but it also can ache physically. By naming and taming your feelings, you also take notice of how your body is holding up against the pressure of life. So, that crick in your neck is not necessarily because of My Pillow, and that lingering headache behind your eye is probably not because it's going to rain tomorrow. When you're stressed, your body pays the price. Now you can notice pains earlier and take the right action.

Mindfulness soothes your lizard brain. Stress responses reside in the amygdala, the caveman-era part of our brain that signals *danger, danger* and tells us to climb a tree or grab a spear. Being mindful calms the crazy from this primitive lizard brain and reminds us that when Mildred and Mary come to visit, the only real threat is to the clean air in the bathroom. Mindfulness also presses the pause button on those racing thoughts and bad coping mechanisms. (*What if they ruin my Eileen Fisher sheets? Oh, my God, I better remember where I hid the cigs.*) You can then use your "wise mind" to come up with better responses. (*Maybe they can babysit so hubby and I can go out.*)

Mindfulness switches you out of your D mode. D mode is your Doing mode, and that's also a Default mode for most of us (after all, nobody gives out prizes for sitting around). But when your mind is always set on doing, producing, and going, going, going, you are primed for stress, stress, stress. Mindfulness requires we activate our B mode — just Being. We learn to live in the Now, to step back and let the world run without our hands on it for a few minutes. As a stress reducer, B mode is highly Beneficial.

And yet . . . mindfulness lets you do more! Anxiety—a reaction from our lizard brain—is an expert liar. It is an overestimation of risk and underestimation of coping ability.

Whether the stressor is an upcoming job interview or six red lights on the way to work, anxiety signals that *You have a big, big problem and you must do something NOW!* It's the mind's equivalent of being thrown in the water when you can't swim: You react, you don't think. You believe the more you thrash around the better off you'll be.

Mindfulness enables you to see the truth of *what is.* It tells you, *slow down, you got this.* It allows you to gather yourself up, step back, take a breath, and reassess. And when you are calm, cool, collected, and not ordering a white chocolate mocha Frappuccino, you think clearly. You see your priorities and act with purpose, not react with impulse. Pretty soon you're the one getting it all done. Hello, Bionic Woman!

For more benefits of mindfulness practices, I recommend Susan Smalley and Diana Winston's book *Fully Present: The Science, Art, and Practice of Mindfulness.*

Christine's Fave Mindfulness Tools

As a mindfulness practitioner for over nine years in the master class at UCLA Mindful Awareness Research Center, I have two favorite go-to stress relief tools: RAIN and STOP.

1) Let it RAIN.

This first tool supports the idea that if you can name it, you can tame it. Created by Michele McDonald, a leading expert in mindfulness meditation, RAIN can be used anywhere, anytime to help you quickly assess what's happening inside.

R: Recognize. Name whatever emotion is coming up for you. *I feel disappointed/ angry/betrayed/hurt/sad.*

A: Allow. Let yourself feel the feeling. Don't judge it; don't beat yourself up for it. If you feel sad, throw on some Gloria Estefan and cry your heart out.

I: Investigate. Check in to see where this feeling comes up in your body. Does your sadness feel like a weight on your chest or an elephant on your shoulders? Is your mind racing faster than Seabiscuit? Are you craving something salty or sweet? Bringing awareness to what you're feeling will allow *you*—not your lizard brain—to choose the response.

N: Not-identify. Now we're tackling the Big Lebowski. Instead of taking your molehill of a feeling and climbing it like Everest *(I ate a cupcake, ergo, I'm a disgusting blob),* you simply choose *not to identify* as your feeling. There's a difference between having a thought and being a thought. *I feel like a loser* does not mean you *are* a loser, any more than saying *I feel like Gwyneth Paltrow* means that you are having sex with ex–Chris Martin.

Here's my favorite technique for Not-Identify. Imagine your mind as a vast blue sky. Imagine your thoughts as vaporous clouds, all shapes and sizes, some devastating, some beautiful, all drifting past. Notice them, admire them, then let them float away, making room for clarity and calm. Remember that passing-by is the natural course of clouds and thoughts. It's only when we to hold onto them that we get stuck.

EMBRACE THE "GOOD" STRESS

Just as we consume bad fats and good fats, we experience "good" stress and "bad." Some stressors—a major operation, sickness, divorce—will always knock us for a loop and require serious attention to our minds, bodies, and emotions. Other stressors—a new job, a visit from Mary and Mildred, a business trip—are actually a gift. Exposure to stress that we can overcome can provide us with higher self-esteem, more resilience, less fear, and more wisdom. Think of that stress as the emotional avocado of our life, filled with super nutritious goodness. So, don't cower away from sucky circumstances, and certainly don't collapse into a bad habit because you think you can't handle your feelings in the moment. If you succeed just one time in responding more positively as a response to your stress, you will start a ripple effect of better responses in the future. If you did it once, you can do it again. It's that simple.

2) Make it STOP.

STOP is another great tool for using in the moment, particularly when someone or something has really pushed your buttons (Los Angeles traffic, anyone?). Essentially, it allows you to pause and *choose* your response before you start making unpleasant gestures out the window. It's a two-minute process that you can do in the car, at the checkout counter, before a big meeting. Thousands of my clients have used it to ramp down stress reactions and make wiser choices.

I love how Holocaust survivor and psychologist Viktor Frankl wrote about coping with a stress response. "Between stimulus and response there is a space," he wrote. "In that space is our power to choose our response. In our response lies our growth and our freedom."

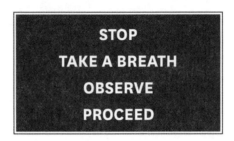

S: Stop. Mentally pause from whatever you're doing, even for a second or two. If someone cuts in line at the coffee shop, just *stop*.

T: Take a breath. Bring your attention back to your breath. Don't try to change it; just notice it. Is it in your chest, your nose, your belly? Your breath is the anchor for you in the moment.

O: Observe. Check in. Are you experiencing any physical sensations or tension? What do you notice about your surroundings? Maybe you'll see that the guy who cut in front of you was innocently distracted or is trying to deal with a cranky kid.

P: Proceed. Return to your activity. Use your new awareness to choose a response. Maybe you're fine letting the situation slide—or maybe you'll call out the cutter with a respectful "Excuse me; the line is behind me." Either way, you're choosing from a place of calm, not chaos!

Christine's Fave Calming Techniques

When the shite hits the fan, your blood rushes to your head and you need to find your footing, *calming* is key. Otherwise, you risk going off the rails and into the depths of Negativeville, where nothing good ever happens and nobody comes out alive. Here are some strategies to keep you centered and on track for your preferred destination: Itsallgood City.

Calming Tool #1: Grounding

Perfect for when a wave of major anxiety is washing over you (if only I'd had this technique on that horrible Bronx River Parkway bus ride). Grounding helps you feel safe in your own head and body when the world around seems crazy.

1) Think of a peaceful place. Use five adjectives, from your five senses, to describe it. *I feel the warmth of the sun, smell the breeze, taste the salty air, hear the squawk of gulls, see a sparkling wave.* (Can you guess where I went in my head?)

2) Picture your most nurturing figures. *I envision Mother Teresa, my friend Louise, and my mindfulness teacher, Diana Winston.*

3) Picture your protective figures. *I think of my dad, my husband, and my grandmother.*

4) Picture three wise figures and remember why you love their philosophies. *I think of Don Miguel Ruiz, Joel Osteen, and my therapist.*

All these images will ground you in your values and remind you of the ways in which you want to live your life. What would these people say, do, advise? How would your favorite place nurture, heal, or revitalize you? Use that space and wisdom to create a better response to your stress.

Calming Tool #2: Rebalancing

When you need to get out of your head STAT, use this technique to counteract those racing thoughts. Ready? Here it is: name six things. That's it. Could be six colors, six breeds of dogs, six songs from Bon Jovi's *Slippery When Wet*, six characters in *Dirty Dancing*. Or if you're going for *major* distraction, go for the whole cast of *Grease* or all of Kevin Bacon's films! It's similar to what you do when your four-year-old is having a hissy fit in the cereal aisle. Divert, pivot, distract—it works!

You'll be rebalanced in a heartbeat.

Calming Tool #3: Acceptance and Equanimity

They're a mouthful, but these concepts saved my life and my sanity. Because I'm an impatient Leader personality prone to Bigger, Better, Faster, and I'll-Be-Happy-When-Syndrome, I needed to learn the concept of *it is what it is*. Buddhists believe that desire is the source of all unhappiness, and it's hard to argue that. But given that we're all human (even if Buddhist), I'd say it's more realistic to simply *stop wanting something to be different from what it is.*

Acceptance and equanimity (which is the understanding that things simply are as they are) teach you to get your ego out of the way, because it's not all about you. *You* are not in control of everything. Moreover, if your boss just fired you, jelly Munchkins are not going to undo that. You gain peace when you learn to work with reality as it is, rather than fight it or feed your face because of it.

For me, accepting *what is* feels extremely freeing. ("If you want less stress, make *isness* your business," says life coach Marie Forleo. Amen!) Once when I was freaking out over a major dental procedure, my teacher (Elisha Goldstein, author of *Uncovering Happiness*) told me, "Your feelings are already here." All I had to do was put out the welcome mat!

For practicing Acceptance and Equanimity, here's a short and sweet exercise from mindfulness teacher Jack Kornfield:

> *Sit in a comfortable posture with eyes closed. Bring soft attention to your breath until body and mind are calm. Reflect on the benefit of a mind that has balance and equanimity. Sense what a gift it can be to bring a peaceful heart to the world around you. Let yourself feel an inner sense of balance and ease. Then begin repeating such phrases as, "May I be balanced and at peace." Acknowledge that all created things arise and pass away: joys, sorrows, pleasant events, people, buildings, animals, nations, even whole civilizations. Let yourself rest in the midst of them. "No matter how I might wish things to be otherwise, things are as they are." "May I learn to see the arising and passing of all nature with equanimity and balance. May I be open and peaceful." "May I one day accept myself just as I am."*

For more on this practice, see Byron Katie's book *Loving What Is: Four Questions That Can Change Your Life.*

Calming Tool #4: Gratitude

This one may give you pause. Because, really, when life throws you a crap boss or car theft, what is there to be grateful for?

To which I say, listen to Robert Emmons, author of *The Little Book of Gratitude:* "It's easy to feel grateful when life is good. But when disaster strikes, gratitude is worth the effort." Why? Because when we are grateful, Emmons says, we get to view life in its entirety and not be overwhelmed by temporary circumstances. We remember the good we had before and look forward to the good that will come again. In fact, Emmons's research at UCLA Davis showed that people who practiced gratitude actually became more resilient against stress.

So the next time you're feeling like it's a dog-eat-dog world and you're wearing Milk Bone underwear (to quote Norm from *Cheers)*, try this gratitude meditation.

> *Settle yourself in a relaxed posture. Breathe deeply and relax. Let your aware-ness move to your immediate environment: all the things you can smell, taste, touch, see, hear. Say to yourself: "For this, I am grateful."*

> *Next, bring to mind those people in your life to whom you are close: your friends, family, partner. Say to yourself, "For this, I am grateful."*

> *Next, turn your attention to yourself: your uniqueness, your imagination, your ability to learn from the past and plan for the future, your ability to overcome any pain you may be experiencing. Say to yourself: "For this, I am grateful."*

> *Finally, rest into the realization that life is a precious gift. That you have been born into a period of immense prosperity, that you have the gift of health, cul-tures and access to spiritual teachings. Say to yourself: "For this, I am grateful."*

Calming Tool #5: Loving Kindness

This is a great one for people-induced stress. Use it when the waiter brings you a steam-ing bowl of tripe instead of your vegan salad; when a coworker snorts instead of blowing his nose; when the gal on the subway has an F-bomb conversation on speakerphone. Loving kindness reminds you that the world is not yours alone nor here to serve you. We are all connected, and loving kindness is a great tool to tone down your ego and keep your stress from tainting your values. (P.S. It's also great when you're in a Kick-Me mood. Don't you deserve loving kindness?)

Created by my teacher Diana Winston of the UCLA Mindful Awareness Research Cen-ter, the Loving Kindness Meditation goes as follows:

> *Let yourself be in a relaxed and comfortable position. We're going to do the practice of cultivating loving kindness, which is the desire for someone to be happy or yourself to be happy. It's not dependent on something, it's not condi-tional. It's just a natural opening of the heart to someone else or to yourself.*

Let yourself bring to mind someone whom, the moment you think of them, you feel happy. It could be a relative, a close friend, a pet; someone with not too complicated a relationship—just a general sense, that when you think of them you feel happy. Have a sense of them being in front of you—you can feel them, sense them, see them. And as you imagine them notice how you're feeling inside. Maybe you feel some warmth, a smile, sense of expansiveness.

This is loving kindness. This is a natural feeling that's accessible to all of us at any moment. So now having this loved one in front of you, begin to wish them well. "May you be safe and protected from danger. May you be happy and peaceful. May you be healthy and strong. May you have ease and wellbeing."

Now imagine that this loved one turns around and begins to send it back to you. Take it in. Now if it's possible, and it's not always easy to do this at first, see if you can send loving kindness to yourself." You can imagine it coming down your body from your heart. You can just have a sense of it and here are some phrases you can offer yourself. "May I be safe and protected from danger. May I be healthy and strong. May I be happy and peaceful."

Calming Tool #6. Self-Compassion

All mindfulness practitioners agree: self-compassion is the single most important tool to combat stress. Loving ourselves, understanding ourselves, and forgiving ourselves are probably the most difficult acts a human can accomplish, which is why this self-compassion tool has been a lifesaver for countless people. As soon as you cut yourself a little slack, you start to feel a little easier in your skin, a little more competent, a little more able to just *deal*. So when your KFKD classics are turned up to 10, give yourself a deep, heartfelt *atta-girl* with this meditation.

Stand, sit, or lie down comfortably. Take a few deep breaths and feel free to put your hand over your heart. Follow your hand rising and falling on your chest. You may take a mental note for whatever difficulty is coming up for you. A fight with a coworker, disagreement with family, a mistake you feel frustrated with. Just let whatever arises be there without judgment. Allow yourself to know that difficult emotions come and go just like a wave in the ocean.

Allow yourself some kind phrases: "I care about your suffering." "For whatever it is I am feeling, may I hold this with kindness. May I love myself just as I am." "For any harm I may have caused myself, knowingly or unknowingly, through my thoughts, words, and actions, I offer my forgiveness as best I am able."

And finally . . .

Don't sweat it. Really. Whatever form your stress takes, know that others have faced it, as well. You. Are. Not. Alone! Allow yourself to know that, today, you get to choose to *respond* instead of *react*. And allow yourself to try all of these meditations and see what feels like a Right Fit for you. Don't worry if your mind still wanders or you don't "get" it—there's a reason it's called a practice!

Here's the thing. As the Queen of NYC Neurosis, I used to view life through a metaphorical soda straw, seeing nothing but perceived shortcomings, mine and everyone else's. Mindfulness gave me a wide-angle lens. I see myself now as I am, strengths, emotions, and all. I see my life as a series of opportunities and gifts, not just a series of problems and challenges. It really works! So allow these ideas and exercises to make you loud and proud of your newfound resilience. Or at the very least, a whole lot calmer!

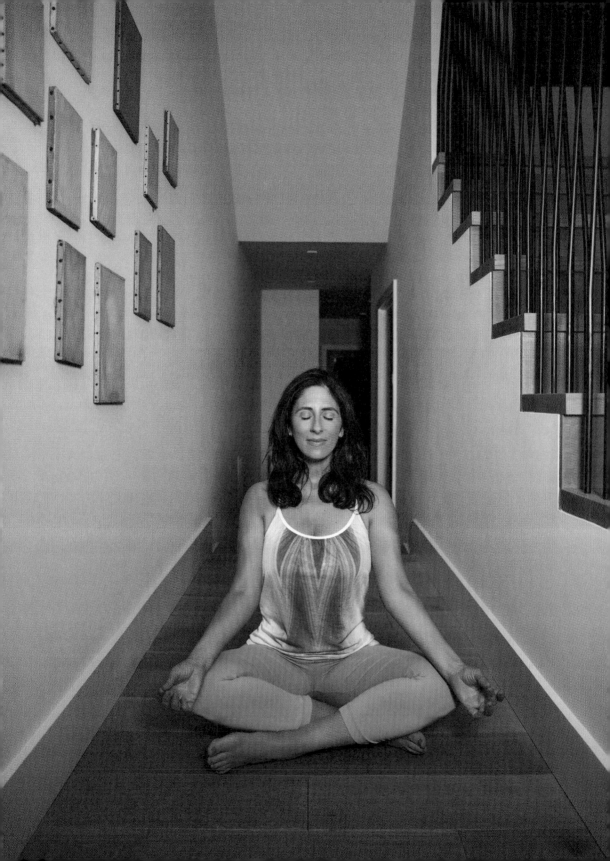

Match Dot CALM

Every personality has a different kind of crazy, and every personality has a different kind of calm. While the above practices are great for nearly everyone, it's nice to check in with *your* kind of stress management. As always, feel free to mix and match because it's likely you are a mixed bag, too!

Leaders

Your kind of crazy: Impatience! You like control and want to handle situations with your own resources and inner wisdom. But when a WTF situation comes up, watch out! Your inner wisdom gets clouded, you can't think, and so you *react*. (Which is when coworkers quake in their cubicles!)

Your kind of calm: You need quick and effective. This Body-Scan Meditation, from the UCLA Mindful Awareness Research Center, takes less than three minutes and provides clarity. Welcome back, inner wisdom and *sanity!*

> *Begin by bringing your attention into your body. You can close your eyes if that's comfortable to you. You can notice your body, seated: feeling the weight of your body on the chair, on the floor. Take a few deep breaths, and as you take a deep breath, bring in more oxygen and liven the body. And as you exhale, have a sense of relaxing more deeply. You can notice the sensation of your feet touching the floor: the weight and pressure, vibration, heat. You can notice your legs against the chair: pressure, pulsing, heaviness, lightness. Notice your back against the chair. Bring your attention into your stomach area. If your stomach is tense or tight, let it soften. Take a breath. Notice your hands—are your hands tense or tight? See if you can allow them to soften. Notice your arms; feel any sensation in your arms. Let your shoulders be soft. Notice your neck and throat; let them be soft, relaxed. Soften your jaw. Let your face and facial muscles be soft. Then notice your whole body present. Take one more breath. Be aware of your whole body, as best you can. Take a breath. And then when you're ready, you can open your eyes.*

Socializers

Your kind of crazy: Tilt-a-Whirl! You're going in five different directions at once, asking everyone except yourself for answers and insight. Trust yourself to handle that overdue report or that meddling in-law? Never!

Your kind of calm: Groundedness. Try this Mountain Meditation from psychologist Peter Morgan to gain control over your reactions to stress. (This is adapted; for the full meditation, visit freemindfulness.org.)

Allow the mountain to remind you of the resiliency that resides within you.

> *Find a comfortable and quiet place to sit with your back straight. Close your eyes and take three deep and slow breaths. Continue breathing slowly from the base of your spine to your heart. As you breathe in, imagine you are breathing in the strength and resiliency of a mountain. As you breathe out, imagine you can weather any storm, freezing rain, snow, the hot summer. Day and night, you are rooted and unwavering in your stillness, just like the mountain. Repeat this breath cycle for ten minutes or more.*

. . . .

Supporters

Your kind of crazy: Frustration! While you're a pretty cool customer by nature, chaos and unpredictability can throw you off fast. If you've got a day of thwarted routines—a flat tire, a late bus, your favorite restaurant closed by the Health Department—you need to decompress, and without the Cheetos, please.

Your kind of calm: A Walking Meditation is perfect. You'll feel calmer, but you'll also feel that sense of "doing." I mean, you can't just *sit* there!

> *Select a quiet place where you can walk comfortably back and forth, indoors or out, about ten to thirty paces in length. Plant your feet firmly; let your hands rest easily. Open your senses to see and feel your surroundings. Feel how your body is standing on the earth. Let yourself be present and alert.*

> *Begin to walk a bit more slowly than usual. Let yourself walk with a sense of ease and dignity, as if you were a king or queen out for a royal stroll. With each step feel the sensations of lifting your foot and leg off of the ground. Then mindfully place your foot back down. When you reach the end of your path, pause for a moment. Center yourself, carefully turn around, pause again so that you can be aware of the first step as you walk back. Continue to walk back and forth for five or ten minutes or longer. If you like, use phrases to bring your mind to attention. You can say "lifting" and "placing" or use inspirational phrases with each step, such as these from the Thich Nhat Hanh's poem, "I Have Arrived": "I am free, I have arrived, I am solid, I am home."*

Planners

Your kind of crazy: Perfectionism! When the recipe doesn't work . . . when the numbers don't crunch . . . when the data is a dump . . . well, you're just not a happy camper, and you just *know* there's a Dove bar nearby calling your name.

Your kind of calm: You're not going to like this, but: Let. It. Go. Stop playing God (who is in the details) for a few minutes and check out the Letting-Go Meditation below. The sooner you release your expectations of how things *should* have happened, the sooner you'll find the calm and resilience to back away from the treats in the freezer.

> *Sit in a comfortable position; focus on your breathing for a few minutes and settle into a calm space. Think about the different parts of your body: skin, blood, bones, organs. Think how each part is in turn made up of veins, cells, tendons—things we can't see but know they work; know that they are moving, changing, reproducing, dying. Consider how you've changed from a young child to now.*
>
> *Now take that awareness outside yourself. The earth and trees, flowers, clouds, buildings, all come and go. They are not static nor frozen but constantly moving and changing, every second, every day.*
>
> *Now think about what you may be holding onto that reminds you of what you didn't want to have change. Consider your belief that things should be a certain way and then the reality that change is the only constant in life. Try squeezing your hand tightly. Notice tension that occurs when we're holding on tightly. Notice what it feels like to be "caught." Now open your palm and notice what it feels like to let go. Feel the sense of ease and peace and release.*

. . . .

I'll leave you with these thoughts by meditation master Ajahn Chah. "If you let go a little you will have a little peace; if you let go a lot you will have a lot of peace; if you let go completely you will have complete peace."

Amazing how three little words (Let-it-go) lead to immense happiness.

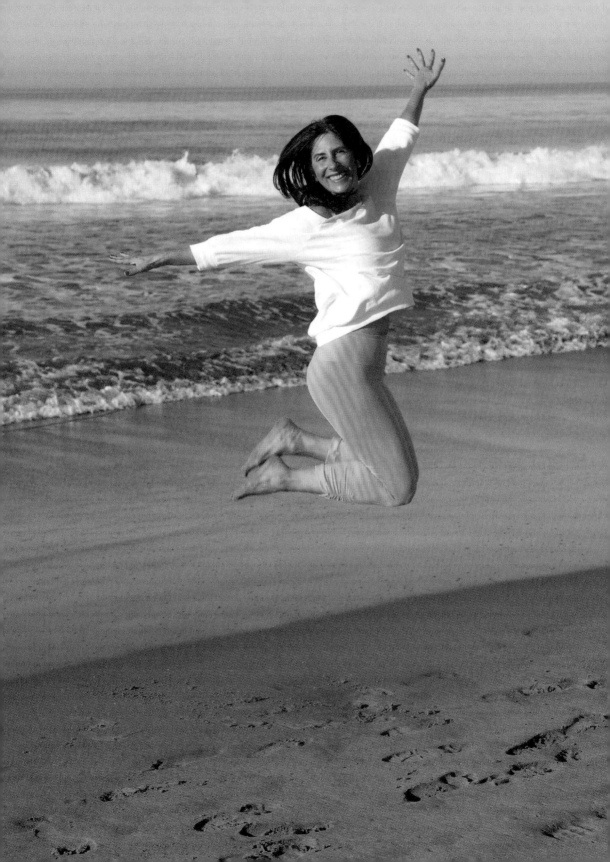

CHAPTER ELEVEN

Let's Get Physical!
(The Day Has Finally Come)

■■■

Welcome to Your Least Favorite Chapter!

IF I KNOW YOU—and I think I do—the word "workout" probably sounds to you the way "flea bath" sounds to a cat. *You don't wanna exercise!* I get it! You've done it all before, it was hard, it sucked, and worst of all, *it didn't work.* Am I right?

Okay. Now dry your tears, hitch up your big-girl pants, and listen while I clue you in as to why exercise has been at the top of your shit list, and why it's about to come off.

Here's the reason you hated exercise: *you wanted to lose weight.*

Well, duh! What's wrong with that?

Here's what's wrong: When we exercise for weight loss—*purely* for weight loss—we go hardcore, and we make choices that are completely out of alignment with who we are. We grit our teeth and tough it out. We do treadmills, boot camp, CrossFit, circuit training, anything that promises to burn half-a-day's calories in an hour. We hate pretty much every second, but we do it. Hey, I've been there: I was the crazy lady doing triple sessions on the StairMaster, remember?

But guess what happens when we do something we hate. We avoid it. We find excuses, we show up late, and soon we don't show up at all. At that point, we tell ourselves it didn't work, woe is me, and let's see what's on Netflix.

But of course we know that exercise *does* work. It works if we do it consistently. But we only do it consistently when we enjoy it and see results.

So here's why exercise is about to come off your shit list: *You're going to approach it from the inside-out instead of the outside-in.*

In other words, you're *not* going to work out strictly for some outer goal, like "lose 10 pounds" or "get a sexy booty." Instead, you're going to work out for *fun.* You're going to explore what feels good to your body and makes sense to your mind. You're going to treat exercise like play instead of work. No maxing out, no counting reps, no whip at your back. Don't get me wrong: if you keep at it, you *will* lose weight and get a hotter booty! But *the only way you'll keep working out is if you love working out.* So let's feel the love!

Epiphany on the Beach (Thanks, Jay!)

Of course, I had to find all this out the hard way. One day, while I was in the middle of Yo-Yo Dieting Session No. 135, I spent an afternoon running on the beach with my husband, Jay. And I was having one of *those* days. No energy, a horrible mood, and a mind full of friends' divorces, unpaid bills, endangered white rhinos, you name it. After I huffed and grunted through an entire half-marathon (okay, it was five miles, but I could swear it was more), I finally caught up with Jay, who was not only huff-less, but *smiling.* What the—?

He told me I looked miserable. I responded, with as few curse words as possible, *Yes, I'm miserable! I ran five miles, and this is the $%#& best mood I could get?* He then told me something—God bless him—that made perfect, instant sense. "Being physical is going to be a part of our lives forever," he said. "It's essential. So you have to make this easier on yourself, Christine, not harder."

Eureka! I never, ever considered making things *easier* for myself.

Until that moment, my whole concept of exercise was that every session had to be tougher than the one before. Challenge yourself, right? Wrong. That day, I adopted a new workout mantra: *If it feels good, it matters. If it doesn't feel good, it's nothing.* If I'm clearing my head with a five-minute yoga inversion, it matters. If I'm enjoying a five-mile hike with my dog, it matters. If I'm gasping through a five-mile run and I'm just not feelin' it, it's punishment. It's not worth it.

From that day on, I set up my exercise program to succeed, not fail. These days, I check in with myself: What's my energy level? What's my mood? Sometimes I want to blow off steam with big-time cardio. Sometimes I want a stretchy, slow Pilates session. Sometimes I just want to dance my butt off. **Whatever it is I am feeling, I honor it with one big goal in mind:** *to feel good.*

And, guess what: I still love running on the beach, *when I feel like it.* I just don't do the misery part! Let me share with you what I've learned on this journey, and I'll help you explore what kind of workout matters for *you.*

Christine's Exercise Wisdom: Five Easy Pieces

Before we get to actually moving our bodies, let's work on our minds. You'll get the most out of your workout—whichever workout you choose—if you adopt the following concepts:

1. Move with purpose

I'm not crazy about the terms "exercise" and "working out." They sound chore-like, necessary, and boring, sort of like doing laundry and loading the dishwasher.

These days, I prefer to say *movement with purpose.* I want to tattoo this on my arm because it's my own personal belief system for everything I do, not just working out. If something doesn't make sense to me, I just won't do it! And if something *does* make sense, and feels like it supports my values and goals, then I do it, and with purpose.

Movement with purpose also means that any time I'm moving my body, I make sure it matters. Whether it's walking the dog or doing back extensions, whatever movement I choose has to feel good right then and there for where I am that day. I'm done with so-called "exercise"—that stuff you push through in order to get it over with. These days I'm all about doing what feels right. Which leads me to this . . .

2. Try Radical Acceptance

I love this concept created by author Tara Brach. Radical Acceptance is simply this: you accept yourself as you are while also moving forward. It's "radical" because most of us believe that we need to reject our "bad" parts in order to change. If you accept yourself, why change? And if you want to change, doesn't that mean you don't like something about yourself? Actually, no. Radical Acceptance means that you fully embrace who you are—all your history, your sufferings, your joys, your choices. What emerges from that acceptance is a calm, peaceful state of being. You begin to love yourself enough to move on, rather than beat yourself up for eating that piece of cake, skipping your workout, or choosing the wrong job. You don't have to hate yourself to change: in fact, the only way to change is to accept yourself while making strides in the direction of what you desire and value.

3. Play, don't work

Yes, I mean this literally. When you start exploring workouts, you're going to go for the ones that will not feel like work. Just pick five to try this month, three days a week. (I'll give some ideas below.) After completing each session, ask yourself these questions:

Was it fun?
Does my body feel good?
Am I smiling?
Would I like to do it again?
Am I looking forward to improving?
Do I feel good about what I accomplished?
Has my mood changed?

Write down which workouts left you smiling:

1) _____
2) _____
3) _____
4) _____
5) _____

I want you to keep this list close, and remember: when time is short and stress is high, *these workouts made you smile.* You may think you have 14 excuses why you just *can't* do it today (and we'll also get to those excuses in a moment), but when you remember how good you felt doing that kickboxing or that yoga class, you will know that you are worth every ounce of time and effort.

4. Outthink your excuses

Joey was my most attitudinally challenged client ever. He liked to party, he liked cigars, and he did not like to move with purpose unless it was to the refrigerator for a beer. His wife, terrified that he would have a heart attack, gave him *me* as a birthday present!

So every Monday, while totally hurting from the weekend's festivities, Joey would give me every excuse in the book as to why he hadn't worked out. *I had a company party. My kids were up all night. We had to meet with clients.* We made a deal: he could give me any excuse he wanted, and once we wrote it down, he was forbidden from using it again.

The longer Joey's excuse list got, the more he could see it for the BS that it was. The truth was that he was stressed and he was dealing with it by partying. So after we finally got him on the treadmill, I guided him into noticing his breath, his thoughts (were they supporting or resisting?), and his physical sensations. Before long, his competitive streak kicked in (he was a hard-driving Leader type, of course), and he started seeing how much he could push. When it was over, Joey was . . . smiling! "I can't believe I did that!" he said. "I haven't been able to run like that since my twenties!"

Being the Leader he was, Joey went all in. He started a company softball team, and—cue uplifting movie music—six months after beginning his training, he placed first in his age group at a fundraiser half-marathon! The video alone defies logic: this out-of-shape curmudgeon became a confident champion.

If, like Joey, you find yourself in one of those "Sorry, not today" moods, try writing your own excuse list. See if you can separate the real reasons (just broke my leg, baby has croup, 500-page report due tomorrow) from the smokescreens (just broke my nail, husband has a cold, have to finish this memo). Then take a cue from Spike Lee and do the right thing!

Your Excuses

1) _____

2) _____

3) _____

4) _____

5) _____

5. Cash in on the benefits!

Here's something I left out of Joey's story: after six months of working out, he found, to his amazement, that his job and family were so much less annoying!

And no, he hadn't switched jobs *or* families. He switched attitudes. The healthier Joey got, the more focused he became at work and the more patient he became at home.

And Joey, I have to say, is just one of hundreds of people I've seen whose lives have been changed by fitness.

Allow me to thump the Bible for just a minute. Physical fitness is an entry point to your best self. Yes, it builds endorphins, and endorphins make you feel pleasure and contentment. Yes, it relieves stress. But it also builds resiliency, confidence, and competence. Ask anyone who's completed a marathon. Heck, ask anyone who's completed a 5K! When you tackle something you're afraid of, or when you push yourself a little further than you think you can go, you expand yourself. You build your capacity to stretch, to live with discomfort, to make choices that are a little tougher but a lot more rewarding.

So no, working out is not just about weight loss! When you work out, you are literally building your best life.

Take some time to really explore the information in this chapter. Remember, I'm all about flexibility and options. You'll find the right way of moving that will suit your lifestyle and personality, and I'm pretty sure you'll even have—yes, I'll say it—some fun.

YOUR WORKOUT: CUSTOMIZE IT!

Different moods, different personalities, different workouts! Here's a list of what works for most people and most moods. See which ones could make *your* Go Plan. Notice that I'm staying away from calorie counting; the point is to move with purpose, not to tick off a number. Remember: your workout only matters if it feels good!

Running

Best for when you're feeling: Stressed. It's a great way to unwind, declutter your thinking, and kick in endorphins fast.

Other benefits: Building tolerance to discomfort, building consistency, building confidence.

Often chosen by: Leaders (that competitive streak!), Supporters (easy way to check out the neighborhood), and Socializers (if friends are going, too!).

Pilates

Best for when you're feeling: Unfocused or chaotic. With its deliberate, focused movement, Pilates connects your mind and body to perform in the present moment.

Other benefits: Building flexibility and core strength.

Often chosen by: Planners (they're great at focus!).

Swimming

Best for when you're feeling: Moody and unsettled. The constant, focused movement brings your mind into alignment while giving you stress-relieving cardio.

Other benefits: Fat loss, improved lung capacity, kindness to joint aches and injuries.

Often chosen by: Leaders (if they're going for a personal best) and Planners (who love perfecting strokes and improving times).

Team Sports

Best for when you're feeling: Preoccupied or self-involved. There's no "I" in team!

Other benefits: Bringing out that inner champion and holding yourself accountable for your actions.

Often chosen by: Socializers (especially if everyone's going for a beer later), Leaders (as long as they get to bat first), and Supporters (they know everyone on the team, anyway).

True story: This Leader girl (me) joined a softball team. This Leader girl hated being told where to stand and what to do. So this Leader girl created her own team. Telling others where to stand and what to do? *That* was fun!

Tennis/Squash/Racquetball

Best if you're feeling: Angsty or riled up. Nothing like whacking that ball when you'd like to whack someone's head!

Other benefits: Burning major calories while bringing out that inner Roger Federer.

Often chosen by: Leaders (who love that sense of control and stress relief!) and Planners (who enjoy perfecting strokes and ball control).

Hiking

Best if you're feeling: Overwhelmed or contemplative. Being alone (or with good company) in nature is a wonderful antidote for a tough week.

Other benefits: Sweating without the pounding on your joints.

Often chosen by: Supporters (who love bonding with friends and family), Socializers (ditto), and Planners (who enjoy the opportunity to ruminate).

Cycling

Best if you're feeling: Stressed. Like running, it gives you the endorphin benefits of a nice cardio workout.

Other benefits: Can be done indoors or out, in any season, and you can choose a speed or course to match your mood.

Often chosen by: Leaders (that stress relief) and Supporters (easy way to burn calories while running errands).

Golf

Best if you're feeling: Unfocused. When every move you make is strategic, you simply can't pay attention to (as the Buddhists call it) your drunken-monkey brain.

Other benefits: By transforming mental energy into physical, golf gives you a great transition into sports like baseball.

Often chosen by: Supporters (who are happy playing the same course again and again and again) and Planners (who love analysis and strategy).

Yoga

Best if you're feeling: In need of a fresh start. It's a wonderful exercise for unwinding or starting your weekend or morning.

Other benefits: Improving flexibility, restoring mental sharpness, connecting with your breath and body.

Often chosen by: Supporters (who need the feeling of self-care) and Planners (who enjoy self-evaluation and improvement).

CrossFit/P90X/Circuit Training

Best when you're feeling: Like a big head of steam. These intense sessions push your body to its limits.

Other benefits: Burning major calories, gaining strength and confidence, and tolerating discomfort.

Often chosen by: Leaders (huge stress reliever) and anyone who's young and in good shape already!

Dance/Aerobics

Best when you're feeling: Stressed or low on energy. You get to free your mind and shake your booty.

Other benefits: Burning fat and calories, building cardio strength.

Often chosen by: Socializers (especially if the instructor is hot and you get to rock a cute outfit!).

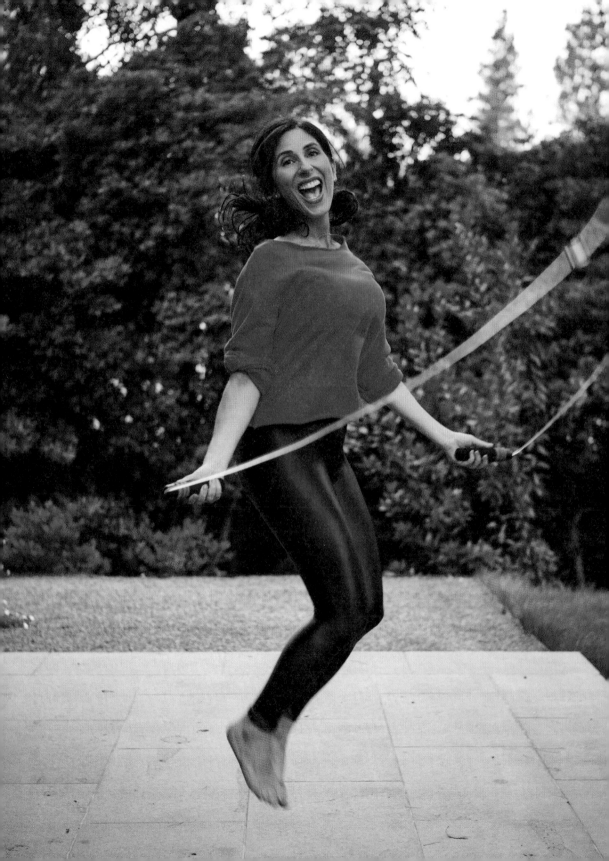

Your Best Life (and Workout) RX

I truly believe that the way you work out reflects the way you live. After all, you're not just training your body. You're training your attitude, your emotional flexibility, and your self-regard. All of that will serve you (or not!) in every aspect of your life.

So let's help you do all of it at your *best*! Based on my decades of experience, I've worked out this prescription for what everyone needs for living (and working out) at his or her peak.

Here's what I share with my clients:

RX No. 1: Do what feels good. Choose activities that are inspiring, energizing, and above all, enjoyable!

RX No. 2: When starting something new, set the bar low. If you've spent the last 20 years in a La-Z-Boy, you're not exactly ready for American Ninja Warrior. But you *can* walk on a treadmill, or around the block! When you start with something you *know* you can do, you build confidence. Confidence gives you the motivation to keep pushing. Every marathon is done one step at a time.

RX No. 3: Schedule a daily and weekly time to work out. Three days a week is a good start, and if it's scheduled, it's likely to get done. Keep it nonnegotiable. Your doctor charges if you miss an appointment, so why should you respect your time any less? Besides, when you do activities that you enjoy, you'll look forward to this time. Refer back to Chapter 5 if you get stuck on where to fit it in.

RX No. 4: But keep your mindset *flexible*. If you set out for your Pilates class but the studio's closed, go home and do a livestream workout, or take the dog on an extralong walk. If you set out to run three miles but poop out after two, celebrate what you did. You won't always be able to give 100 percent, and that's okay. A flexible mindset promotes healthy change; a rigid mindset leads to defeat.

RX No. 5: Celebrate small successes. Everyone does better with an "atta girl." Right after reaching the finish line—wherever the line is that day—use the moment to reflect on how far you've come. I like to finish up with a few simple breaths and open arm stretches. That reflective pause has significantly increased my self-appreciation.

RX No. 6: Track your progress. I never knew how powerful this was until a trainer clocked me running stadium laps years ago. Next time I ran that track, I *really wanted to beat that time.* There is no greater feeling than knowing that you're accomplished and strong, and that stopwatch and exercise log let you know it. But remember . . .

RX No. 7: Any movement is progress. If all you can do is two-thirds of your best time, well, that's still movement, baby. Any time you're moving, you're doing *great.*

RX No. 8: When you compare, you despair. Every time you say, "I wish I had her [whatever]," you give yourself one more little punch to the gut. **It's really hard to change something you don't value.** The more you value what you have, the harder you'll work for it. So praise your body for what it *does* and pay no attention to how hers *looks.*

RX No. 9: Get into action. I swear you could sink a Chinese freighter with the unused dumbbells I've seen in clients' houses. We buy this stuff thinking that the motivation to use it will somehow descend like fairy dust. Sorry, no. Motivation *follows* action. It's when you pick the damn thing up that you actually get the desire to use it. So pick it up! Which means:

RX No. 10: Don't wait for the perfect moment to get moving. It doesn't exist. If all you have are five minutes after the kids leave for school, do jumping jacks! If all you have are 90 seconds while you nuke your lunch, do push-ups against the counter! Remember, everything counts, and it all adds up.

RX No. 11: Combine cardio and strength training. Both are equally effective in weight loss, and they're better together. In fact, adding two or three weekly weight-training sessions (15–20 minutes each) will significantly move the dial on your progress. Moreover, it will help you live longer and stronger. When I'm at the doctor's these days, I love hearing the nurse remark about how low my resting pulse is. Thanks, cardio!

RX No. 12: Intervals, yes! Some days, slow and steady cardio is what your body wants; other days you're ready for a little speed. But if you want to dial it up, try intervals. Intervals combine short sprints of intense cardio (30 seconds to 3 minutes) with rest and recovery of an equal amount of time. Repeat for 15–45 minutes.

Pro tip: For maximum weight loss results, alternate interval workouts with slow-and-steady cardio workouts. It's my secret go-to weapon around the holidays. And it's one of my favorite techniques I've used with Dr. Robert Huizenga. I've worked with patients in his weight loss clinic for 10 years, and it works!

RX No. 13: Give yourself permission to suck at it. For years, I absolutely despised the idea of running. Finally I decided, *fine, I'll just walk around the block*. One block became two, then five. Then I started running a block. Then two. Then five. I loved surprising myself with, *hey, that's not bad. Let's keep going.* Weirdly, giving myself the okay to suck at running got me over my dislike of it. And I discovered I was pretty darn good at it, too!

So if you think you'll stink at tennis, golf, or swimming, you might be right. But you also might be wrong, and it's worth it to start slowly just to see how it feels. You know the mantra by now: if it feels good, *it matters!* And if not, it feels good to have tried.

RX No. Lucky 14: Keep showing up! Consistency is the key to any successful workout routine. Even if (or especially if) you feel like you're wearing lead underwear while swimming through peanut butter, just show up. And remember RX No. 6: Any movement is progress. So move it!

RX No. 15: Become body wise: *Do not push through pain.* There may be certain exercises that just aren't right for your body. *Totally* normal. My body, for instance, hates spinning. My hip flexors hurt no matter how much I adjust the bike, so no, you spin instructors, my form *isn't* wrong—it just hurts. So you know what I do? Forget. About. It. No pain, no pain, people! Go for sensation (stretching or muscle burn), but please avoid pain.

NAME IT AND CLAIM IT

Take a moment to list three goals or intentions you have for getting physical. (Use the SMARTER system in Chapter 8 to help define your choices.)

Then, think about why you want to achieve this particular goal. What's the real reason you want to work out? If your intention is to swim three times a week, for instance, ask yourself: Is this because the pool is convenient (although the chlorine makes you sneeze and the goggles leave you with raccoon eyes for hours)? Or is this because you absolutely love being in the water and want to make more time for it?

I think you know which reason will keep you coming back for more!

1) My goal or intention _____

I want to achieve this because _____

2) My goal or intention _____

I want to achieve this because _____

3) My goal or intention _____

I want to achieve this because _____

Pssst, Over Here! Look Slimmer and Younger Instantly!

If you want the secret of Eternal Youth, check your backside.

You heard me. Somebody should invent glasses with rear-view mirrors—and I mean *rear* as in your butt. Think about it: when you work out, you're looking at your front and occasionally your side. But training your backside has more going for it than just a perky keister. Your booty muscles pretty much rule your posture and gait, from ankle to hip. Yes, your knee or hip pain could be the result of weak glutes! What's more, a little toning of the small back muscles can make you stand straighter and taller and, need I add, make you look 10 pounds lighter.

The rest of your back needs love, too. *This is important, my working-woman friends!* Particularly if you're at the computer all day (and who isn't?), **you need to train your upper back.** Do it, and you'll lose neck tension, improve your posture, age more gracefully (those who stand tall carry themselves more confidently), and put off the day when your back goes out for *no reason.* (Hello? Those atrophied muscles weren't ready for you to rake the lawn!)

Here's a tip from an 80-year-old gent I know with perfect posture and still-killer upper body. Interlock your fingers, place your hands behind your head, and press the back of your head, hard, into your hands (elbows out, eyes ahead) as if you were trying to imprint your skull. Hold for a minute. Let go. Congratulate yourself on gaining an inch in height.

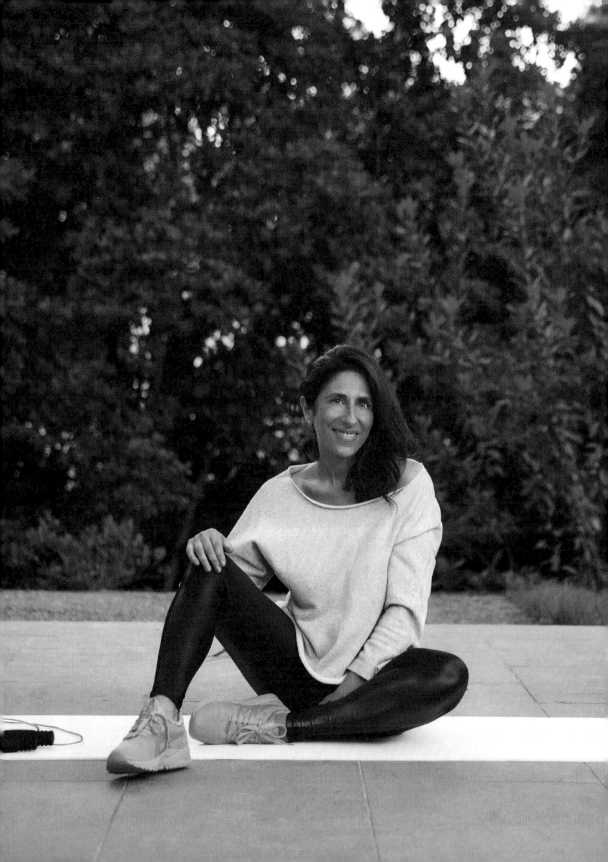

CHAPTER TWELVE

Ding-dong! Your Personal Trainer Has Arrived!

■ ■ ■

Workouts Are Not One-Size-Fits-All.

WELCOME TO YOUR *Right Fit Formula* for exercise. If you're going to move with purpose, that purpose has to make sense to you and feel good. And guess what. I've got a pretty good idea of what's going to make sense *for you.* Having coached many personalities over the years, I know what gets you moving and what keeps you on the couch (I've heard all the excuses, people!). I've selected exercises that I know from experience will fit right in with your personality and lifestyle.

Whether you're a Leader, Socializer, Supporter, or Planner, you'll have six different options to play with, most of which can be done right in your garage or living room.

So let's get those sneakers on and I'll meet you at the mat!

Leader Personality Workout

You, my Leader peeps, are results-oriented. When you work out, you're in it to win it. You might be lifting weights in your garage, but in your head, you're Rocky in a meat locker, punching out sides of beef.

Which is totally great—*if* you're actually working out! The problem with you guys is that you're not spending time in a fantasy meat locker; you're spending it in some real-life drama *du jour.* You've always got another meeting to run, another project to attend to, another fire to be put out somewhere. So you have to trust me when I say these workouts are designed just for you. You'll get in there, crush it, get out, and feel great. Because you run hot, you'll be drawn to the cardio workouts, but try to work in strength and flexibility, as well. Rocky would!

Cardio Workout 1: *HIIT it!*

Duration: 15 minutes
Prop: Flex band.

This High Intensity Interval Training is a simple set of 30-second sequences: 20 seconds at a high-intensity pace followed by 10 seconds of rest. You'll repeat the set of exercises 3 times for a fast, effective 15-minute workout.

Movement 1: Jumping Jacks with band

* Pull band taut between hands, shoulder distance apart.
* Jump out, push band out.
* Jump in, pull band in.
* Repeat for 20 seconds.

Movement 2: Jack Squat with band

* Jump out into squat, band taut, shoulder distance apart, arms lifted.
* Jump in, straighten legs, feet together, lower arms to shoulder distance.
* Repeat for 20 seconds.

Movement 3: Cross Taps with band

* Holding band taut, right leg steps behind you, tapping floor to left.
* Left arm crosses in front of you, tapping floor to right.
* Alternate sides for 20 seconds.

Movement 4: Lateral Leaps (or Steps) with band

* Holding band taut, shoulder height, alternate hops/steps to right and left.
* Repeat for 20 seconds.

Movement 5: Burpees with band

* Holding band taut, jump and reach arms up.
* Squat down, hands to floor, kick legs out to plank position.
* Jump legs forward to squat, stand up.
* Jump, reach arms up.
* Repeat for 20 seconds.

Movement 6: Mountain Climber

* Assume plank position: shoulders over wrists, hips low, core zipped tight.
* Bend right knee toward chest, maintaining low hips and tight core.
* Alternate knees rapidly for 20 seconds.

Movement 7: Repeater Steps with band

* Stand and hold band taut between hands, shoulder height and distance apart.
* Front lunge: step one knee into center and out, 3x.
* Step-back lunge; reach arms out, 3x.
* Step in, reach arms in.
* Repeat for 20 seconds on each leg.

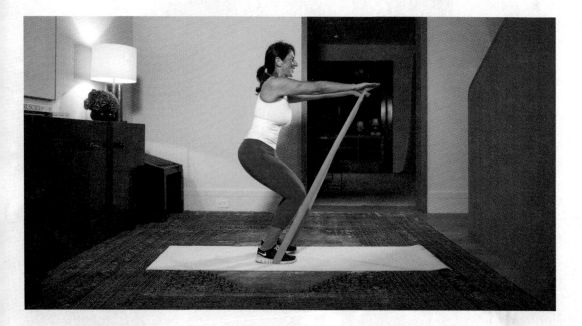

Strength Workout 1: *Flex Band Strength Training*

Duration: 20–30 minutes
Prop: Flex band.

Standing Arm Sequence

Strengthens triceps, biceps, delts, lats, rhomboids, core.

Movement 1: Straight Arms, Lift and Lower
* Standing, place band under feet.
* Hold band with hands, shoulder distance apart.
* With arms straight, pull up against resistance of band.
* Keep small range of motion.
* Repeat double arms 8x.
* Repeat single arm 8x each arm.

Movement 2: Bicep Curls
* Continue with above setup.
* Keep elbows glued to hips.
* Bend elbows slowly and fully against resistance of band.
* Return to starting position with control.
* Repeat double arms 8x.
* Repeat single arm 8x each arm.

Movement 3: Push, Pull, Pulse
* Continue with above setup.
* Keep elbows lifted, arms shoulder height or slightly lower.
* Bend elbows 1 inch, resisting the band.
* Return to starting position.
* Bend and straighten: Push arms forward and pull arms back, keeping arms shoulder height.
* Repeat slow, small range of motion 8x.
* Pulse 8x.

Movement 4: External Rotation
* Stand on band.
* Cross band and hold taut in front of you.
* Palms up, bend elbows to 90 degrees and keep them glued at hips.
* Open forearms wide, externally rotating at the shoulder socket.
* Repeat full range of motion 8x.
* Pulse 8x, holding wide.
* Isolate single arm; repeat 8x.
* Repeat opposite arm 8x.

Movement 5: Tricep Extension

* Continue with above setup as but reverse grip with hands, with ends of band hanging out by pinkies.
* Move right arm slightly behind torso, left hand holding band at waist.
* Bend right elbow slightly, then straighten.
* Repeat full range of motion 8x.
* Pulse 8x.
* Repeat opposite arm.

Repeat above sequence of arm movements 3x.

Standing Leg Sequence

Strengthens quads, glutes, ab/ad, core, hamstrings, lats.

Movement 1: Squats with band

* Stand straight, shoulders over hips.
* Place band under feet, hip distance apart.
* Holding band, raise arms to chest height.
* Squat down, hips back, knees over ankles.
* Repeat full slow range of motion 8x.
* Pulse 8x.

Movement 2: Pliés with band

* Keep torso upright position, feet standing inside band.
* Turn legs out, feet wider than shoulders, knees over ankles, arms raised to chest level.
* Press up to straight legs, then return to plié position.
* Repeat full slow range of motion 8x.
* Pulse 8x.

Movement 3: Lateral Leg Lifts with band

* Stand straight, shoulders over hips.
* Place band under feet, hip distance apart.
* Holding band, place hands at hips.
* Lift right leg out to side, moving slowly against resistance of band.
* Repeat each leg 8x.
* Alternate legs 8x.

Movement 4: Single Leg Reach Down (no band)

* Release band.
* Both feet are parallel position, hip distance apart.
* Stand on right leg; send left leg back while reaching down with a straight left arm to a chair seat or coffee table. (Advanced: aim to touch the floor.)
* Repeat 8x.
* Repeat 8x opposite leg.

Repeat entire leg sequence 3x.

Seated Arm Sequence

Strengthens rhomboids, lats, triceps, delts, core.

Movement 1: Seated W's

* Sit in a straight spine position with straight legs.
* Loop band around edges of feet.
* Hold band with ends hanging out by pinkies.
* Pull arms behind torso, leading with elbow.
* Repeat full range of motion 8x.
* Pulse 8x.

Movement 2: Seated V's

* Sit as above.
* Keep arms straight at your side, slightly wider than hips, in an upside-down V position.
* Pull straight arms behind torso one inch.
* Return to starting position.
* Repeat full range of motion 8x.
* Pulse 8x.

Movement 3: Seated X's

* Sit as above.
* Cross band and hold in front of you.
* Bend elbows, pulling both arms behind you.
* Repeat double-arm pulls 8x.
* Repeat single-arm pulls 8x per arm.
* Pulse double arms 8x.

Repeat above arm sequence 3x.

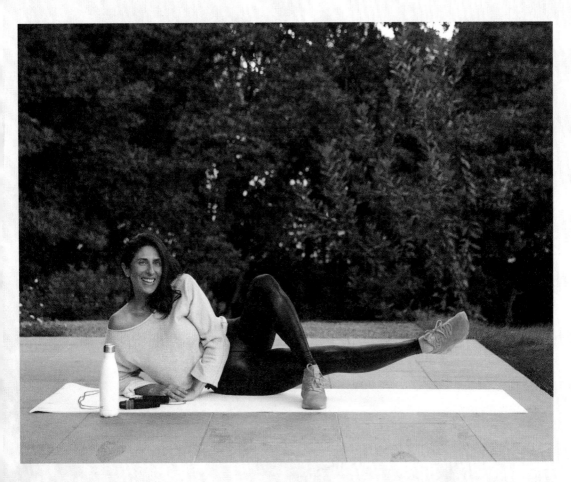

Side Lying Legs Sequence

Strengthens core, lats, outer thighs, glutes.

Movement 1: Side Leg Lift, Parallel
* ⋆ Tie a loop in the band. Place legs in band around base of calf muscles.
* ⋆ Lie on right side, right elbow propped under shoulder, legs straight.
* ⋆ Lift left leg hip height, making sure band offers resistance.
* ⋆ Lift leg higher one inch, then back to starting position.
* ⋆ Repeat 8x.
* ⋆ Pulse 8x.

Movement 2: Forward and Back
* ⋆ Continue in above setup.
* ⋆ Lift leg to hip height.

* Move leg forward one inch, then back to starting position.
* Repeat 8x.
* Pulse 8x.

Movement 3: Side Leg Lift/Turnout
* Repeat Side Leg Lift with toes pointed out.
* Repeat 8x.
* Pulse 8x.

Movement 4: Forward and Back/Turnout
* Repeat Forward and Back sequence with toes pointed out.
* Repeat 8x.
* Pulse 8x.
* Repeat on each leg.

Flexibility Workout 1: *Yoga Stretches*

Prop: Mat or soft surface.

Child's Pose
* Kneel on mat, hips seated over the heels.
* Let chest melt toward thighs. Stretch arms forward, palms down on mat.
* Hold.

Child's Pose Single Side Stretch
* From Child's Pose, reach to left side of mat, maintaining hips over heels.
* Stretch long through the right side. Hold.

Arms Over Head
* Interlace hands behind back.
* Lift arms up, knuckles to ceiling,
* Hold.

Pigeon Hip Stretcher
* In Child's Pose, bring right leg forward with bent knee under your torso.
* Extend left back leg behind you.
* Hold.

Pigeon Quad Stretcher

* ✶ In pigeon, bend left leg up, toes pointing to ceiling.
* ✶ Reach back with left hand and grasp foot.
* ✶ Stretch heel to glute, releasing hip flexor and quad.
* ✶ Hold.

Lat Stretcher

* ✶ In Quad Stretch, release left foot, extending leg long.
* ✶ Extend left hand up and overhead to right side of room.
* ✶ Hold.
* ✶ Push back to Child's Pose.

Repeat sequence on opposite side.

Forward Fold

* ✶ Sit up straight, legs extended in front.
* ✶ Fold forward, releasing hamstrings.
* ✶ Reach arms toward ankles or feet.
* ✶ Hold.

Spinal Twist

* ✶ Sit straight up, legs extended.
* ✶ Bend right knee; cross it over straight left leg.
* ✶ Place left palm on mat behind left hip.
* ✶ Bring right arm across body to hug right knee.
* ✶ Hold twist.
* ✶ Repeat on opposite side.
* ✶ Return to Child's Pose.

Standing Forward Fold

* ✶ From seated position, stand slowly, rounding up one vertebra at a time.
* ✶ Fold forward over thighs, releasing head, shoulders, and neck.

Hip Stretch

* ✶ In Forward Fold, step right leg behind left, lining up baby toes.
* ✶ Reach hands and torso left as you push hips to the right.
* ✶ Repeat opposite side.

Arm and Chest Release

* In forward fold, interlace arms behind back.
* Allow arms to fall over head.
* Now round up to standing, one vertebra at a time.
* Shrug shoulders up, back, forward, and down.
* Stand tall, shoulders over hips, hips over feet, head level.

Cardio Workout 2: *Treadmill Pyramid Intervals*

Duration: 30 minutes
Prop: Treadmill with variable speeds and inclines.

By alternating high- and low-intensity intervals, this workout is designed for max results in minimum time. Adjust speed intensity as needed, but leave inclines as recommended.

Minutes	Speed	Incline
1–5	4	2.0
5–6	5	1.0
6–7	6	1.0
7–8	5	1.0
8–9	6	1.0
9–10	4	1.0
10–11	6.5	1.0
11–12	5	1.0
12–13	7	1.0
13–14	5	1.0
14–15	7.5	1.0
15–16	4	1.0
16–17	6.5	1.0
17–18	5.5	1.0
18–19	7.5	1.0
19–20	5.5	1.0
20–21	8	1.0
21–22	5	1.0
22–23	7	1.0
23–24	5	1.0
24–25	6	1.0
25–30	4	2.0

Strength Workout 2: *Compound Movements with Flex Band*

Prop: Flex band.

Upper Body Sequence

Strengthens core, glutes, shoulders, pecs, lats, balance.

Push-Ups

* ⋆ In push-up position, place inside of band over midback and hold other side with hands firmly to the floor.
* ⋆ Bend both elbows back toward feet.
* ⋆ Push up against resistance of band.
* ⋆ Repeat 8x.

Plank Hold

* ⋆ Continue in above setup.
* ⋆ Keep hips low, in line with the spine.
* ⋆ Hold position to the count of 8.
* ⋆ Extend right arm, holding band.
* ⋆ Hold to count of 8.
* ⋆ Return to plank for 8 counts, then extend left arm for 8 counts.
* ⋆ *Pro tip:* Modify by planking on forearms instead of palms. Place band under elbows.

Tap-out Plank

* ⋆ Continue in above setup.
* ⋆ Lift right leg slightly off floor.
* ⋆ Engage abs for balance.
* ⋆ Tap right leg out 5 inches, then return to center.
* ⋆ Repeat 8x.
* ⋆ Repeat left leg 8x.
* ⋆ Alternate legs 8x.

Pro tip: Modify by planking on forearms instead of palms. Place band under elbows.

Repeat entire sequence 2x

Lower Body Sequence

Strengthens lower body, core, lats, hamstrings, quads; stabilizes spine, improves balance.

Up-Down Leg
* Kneel in tabletop position, hips over knees, shoulders over wrists, spine straight.
* Place band around right foot.
* Place ends of band under hands, holding firmly to floor.
* Extend right leg behind to straight.
* Lift leg up and down, small range of movement, with control.
* Repeat 8x.
* Pulse 8x.

Heel Press to Extension
* Continue in tabletop setup, band around right foot.
* Extend right leg to straight, then return to bend, opening and closing heel to glute.
* Repeat full range of motion 8x.

Alternate
* Alternate Up-Down Leg with Heel Press.
* Repeat 8x.

Small Kick
* Continue in tabletop, band around right foot.
* Keep spine straight, hips level.
* Extend right leg to straight, in line with hips.
* Bend knee softly, one inch, then extend back to straight.
* Repeat 8x, slow.
* Pulse 8x.

Repeat entire sequence 2x. Then repeat entire sequence with opposite leg.

Upper Body Alternate

Strengthens core, triceps, lats, delts; stabilizes spine.

Triceps Kick-Back
* Kneel into tabletop.
* Place left hand on mat under shoulder, holding band firmly to floor.

* Holding band, right hand pulls straight back, brushing right rib cage.
* Bend right elbow, then return to straight.
* Repeat full range of motion 8x.
* Pulse 8x.

Open-Close

* Continue in above setup, right arm holding band, remaining long and straight.
* Move entire arm an inch from center.
* Return to starting position.
* Repeat full range of motion slow 8x.
* Pulse 8x.

Alternate

* Alternate Kick-Backs with Open-Close.
* *Repeat 8x.*

Circles

* Continue in above setup, right arm remaining straight at side.
* Circle right arm slowly with control.
* Repeat 8x in each direction.

Repeat entire sequence 2x. Then repeat series with opposite arm.

Lower Body Alternate

Strengthens core, outer thighs; stabilizes shoulder girdle.

Clam

* Tie a band around thighs just above the knee.
* Lie on side, torso propped on elbow, shoulder over elbow, knees bent 45 degrees.
* As toes remain touching, open knees against resistance of band.
* Open one inch more, then return to start.
* Repeat 8x.
* Pulse 8x.

Parallel Clam

* Remain in above setup.
* Lift top leg to hip height, parallel, feet separated.
* Lift leg one inch more, increasing resistance.
* Return to starting position.
* Repeat 8x.
* Pulse 8x.

Circles

* Remain in above same setup.
* Raise top leg as above.
* Draw large circles with thigh while hips remain stacked.
* Repeat 8x.
* Reverse direction 8x.

Arrow

* Remain in above setup.
* Internally rotate top thigh, bringing knee to floor and toe toward ceiling.
* Press leg up and away from center, increasing resistance.
* Repeat full range of motion 8x.
* Pulse 8x.

Repeat entire sequence 2x. Then switch sides and repeat series.

Flexibility Sequence 2

For this sequence, flex band is doubled between hands. Stand tall with feet slightly wider than hips. Hold each movement 20 seconds.

Side Stretch

* Reach both arms over head, stretching knuckles to ceiling.
* Side bend to right. Hold.
* Side bend to left. Hold.
* Return to straight spine.

Spinal Articulation

* Bend knees, round spine over thighs.
* Straighten legs, bring spine back to straight.

Side Bend Pulls

* With both hands raised, side bend to the right.
* Reach left arm overhead, pulling right elbow to hip.
* Hold.
* Return to center.
* Repeat opposite side.

Wide Plié with Chest Expansion

* Stand in a wide plié stance, feet turned out, knees bent outward.
* Lengthen flex band slightly between hands.
* As right elbow presses right knee open, left arm reaches overhead and slightly behind torso.
* Hold.
* Repeat other side.

Wide Plié with Lat Stretch

* Standing in wide plié, cross left arm in front of torso.
* Pull abs back in opposition.
* Continue to slightly resist with band and press right thigh open.
* Return to center.
* Repeat opposite side.

Cross Stretch

* Straighten legs. Place feet parallel and slightly wider than hips.
* Reach right arm to ceiling, left hand to the floor.
* Hips remain square.
* Hold.
* Repeat opposite side.
* Hold.

Hamstring Stretch

* Lie down on back with one foot on floor.
* Place doubled band around foot on extended leg.
* Connect elbows to floor and press heel up and against band.
* Hold.
* Softly bend knee, then press up again.

* Hold.
* Repeat opposite leg.

Figure 4 Stretch

* Lie on back with feet on floor. Release band.
* Cross right leg over thigh, with knee pointing to right side of room.
* Interlace hands behind left thigh.
* Curl torso up and pull legs to chest.
* Hold.
* Repeat opposite side.

Hip Flexor Release/Quad Release

* Lying on back, place band over hips, low on pelvis.
* Bring heels under knees, arms long at sides, holding band firmly to floor.
* Tuck tailbone under; roll hips up to a shoulder bridge position.
* Lift hips a little higher, feeling stretch in hip flexors.
* Hold.
* Roll down slowly to starting position.

Calf Stretch

* Lying on back, legs extended, place band over balls of both feet.
* Lengthen both legs to ceiling, keeping arms long at side.
* Hold.
* Point and flex feet, both at once and then alternating.

Back Massage

* Lying on back, release band to floor.
* Bend knees into chest and curl into tight ball.
* Rock side-to-side, forward and back.
* Rock to standing position.
* Forward fold.

■■■

Socializer Personality Workout

Hey there! Ready to have some fun? I know you Socializer types: if a workout isn't a good time for you, you're just never going to do it. And for you, a good time means variety, spontaneity, and, if possible, toys. I've got some jump ropes for you, I've got hula hoops, and I've got lots of ideas. It's up to you to crank up the music and shake your booty.

You'll probably enjoy the cardio workout the most, but please don't neglect strength training and flexibility. Combine workouts if you can, but try to get each workout done three times per week.

Pull on your fave leggings and let's get going.

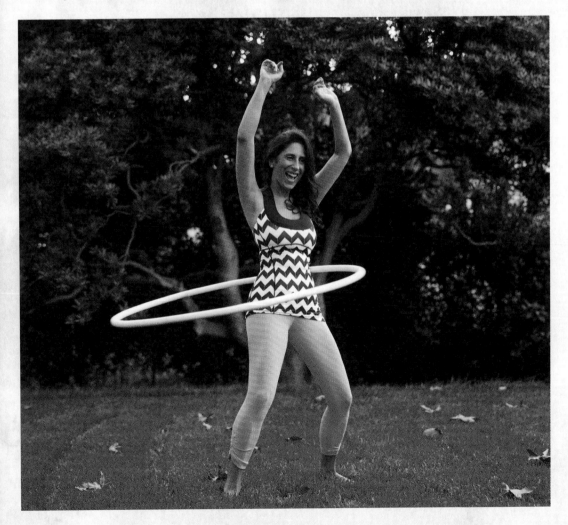

Cardio Workout 1

Props: Exercise hoop, weighing no more than 2 lbs. (Make sure it's designed for adults.) Mat or soft surface.

Hoop It up! Workout: Low Impact, Med/High Intensity Cardio

Duration: 15 minutes

If you're new to hooping, keep at it! It may feel awkward at first, but with time and practice, you'll get better and stay at it longer. All instructions are below. Try to make your hooping intervals as long as possible, but if you get tired, incorporate *lunges and pliés* into your waist-hooping routine. As long as you're moving for 15 minutes, you're golden.

* Hoop for 5 minutes with right leg forward. (To modify, incorporate *right leg lunge-back*.)
* Hoop for 5 minutes with left leg forward. (To modify, incorporate *left leg lunge-back*.)
* Hoop for 5 minutes in a plié stance. (To modify, incorporate *plié sweeps*.)

Higher-Intensity Tips:

* Alternate 1 minute of steady hooping with 2 minutes of hooping as fast as you can. Increase the "fast" duration as you can.
* Add arm movement: punches, arms crossing in front, or arms lowering and lifting overhead.
* Add motion by bending and straightening knees while hooping.

Hooping How-to:

Waist Hooping—Front Stance

* Stand with one foot in front of the other, knees slightly bent, pelvis tucked, torso lifted, head high.
* Place hoop in the small of the back, parallel to ground.
* Give the hoop a strong push with your hand.
* Move hips forward and back.

Lunge-Back

* Standing in parallel, place hoop at right side with right hand on top.

* As you step right leg back into a lunge, roll hoop forward. Check that front knee is over ankle.
* Roll hoop back to your side as you step the right foot back to starting position.
* Repeat for left leg.

Waist Hooping—Plié Stance

* Stand in a plié with feet slightly wider than shoulder distance.
* Knees should be bent softly over the ankles, pelvis tucked, torso lifted.
* Place hoop on the small of the back, parallel to the ground.
* Give the hoop a strong push with your hand.
* Move hips side to side.

Plié Sweeps

* Standing in a wide plié, place hoop in front of you with right hand in center of hoop and left hand extended to the side.
* Lift your right heel high, keeping weight centered.
* Sweep left arm to the right as the right hand rolls hoop to the left, wringing the abdominal wall.
* Return to starting position.

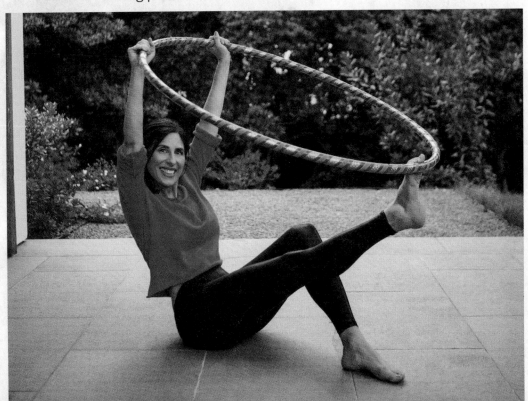

Strength Training: 1—Hoop it Up! Workout

Prop: Hoop, weighing no more than 2 lbs.

Sequence 1: Bodacious Arms

Strengthens deltoids, core, lats and glutes, posture.

Out and In

* Stand in demi-plié: heels together, toes apart, knees slightly bent.
* Hold hoop in front of your chest with hands at 9 and 3. Hands are slightly lower than shoulder height.
* Keeping torso zipped, gently squeeze the sides of the hoop, engaging your pecs.
* With a one-inch range of motion, push arms out straight, then bend elbows and pull back.
* Push and pull for 30 seconds.

Up and Down

* With demi-plié and hands at 9 and 3, bend elbows softly.
* Gently squeeze the hoop between the palms, lifting only the elbows.
* Lift and lower for 30 seconds.

One of Each

* Alternate Out and In and Up and Down for 30 seconds.

Repeat sequence 3x.

Sequence 2: Adding Balance

Strengthens core, deltoids, balance, glutes.

* Stand in demi-plié and hold hoop in front of chest at 9 and 3.
* Tuck pelvis, round spine, and extend right leg behind and slightly to the right, right foot brushing floor.
* Use core for balance as you move hoop through Out and In, Up and Down, and One of Each.
* For added intensity, bend leg in and out while moving arms. Keep range of motion small and precise.
* Repeat each variation 30 seconds.
* Reset and repeat with opposite leg extended.

Pro tip: Balance positions are so important for core strength and stability. Make sure to keep abdominals and glutes engaged to find balance. The extended leg can rest lightly on the floor if needed. Add arm movements only when you find stability in your balance position. Take it one step at a time!

Sequence 3: Plié Pulse

Strengtens glutes, quads, hamstrings, core, calves.

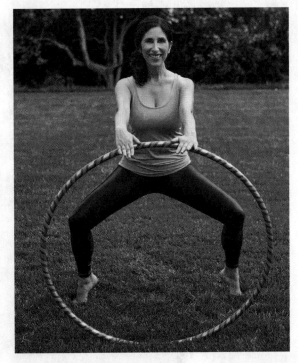

* Place hoop vertically on floor in front of you. Stand in a wide plié, resting hands lightly on top of hoop.
* Keep knees over the ankles and torso upright, shoulders over hips.
* Pulse hips up.
* Repeat 30 seconds.
* Pulse the hips down.
* Repeat 30 seconds.
* Lift right heel high; lift and lower hips one inch.
* Repeat 30 seconds.
* Drop right heel; lift left heel and repeat 30 seconds.

Pro tip: When your quads start to feel fatigue, put your mind into your core muscles. "Zip up" your torso and squeeze glutes to assist.

Sequence 4: Candlestick

Strengthens glutes, abs, hamstrings, stabilizer muscles in the base leg.

* Place hoop vertically at your left, arm's distance away. Rest left hand lightly on top of hoop.
* Bring left knee forward and up to hip level. Point toe; extend right arm in front, shoulder height.
* Hold upright.
* Tip torso forward while extending left leg behind. Right arm lengthens toward the floor.
* Engage your glutes; keep a small, soft bend in standing leg as you maintain torso and leg in straight line.
* Use hoop for light balance as you tip your torso and leg up and down, moving as one unit.
* Bring leg forward. Stand upright.
* Repeat sequence 30 seconds.
* Repeat opposite leg.

Pro tip: Modify the movement by tipping the torso and leg only an inch or two at a time. Your strength, balance, and flexibility will increase with consistency and practice.

Sequence 5: V-ups

Strengthens core, stretches arms and hamstrings, improves breath work.

* Lie on mat with hoop on chest. Keep left foot on ground and place right foot on edge of hoop, right knee bent toward chest.
* Place both hands on the top edge of hoop, shoulder distance apart.
* With arms straight, reach to ceiling. Inhale.
* Exhale as you sit up, extending right leg to straight. The arms and hoop reach up and away from your torso.
* Inhale in upright, seated position; exhale as you lie back down with control. Arms remain straight, right knee bends back into chest.
* Repeat 4x. Switch legs.

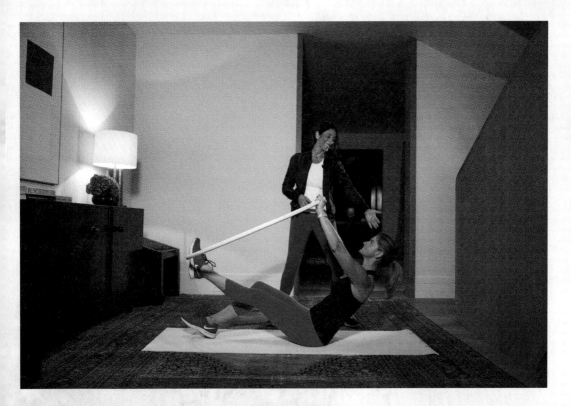

Flexibility Workout 1: *Hoop flow*

Prop: Hoop, weighted with no more than 2 lbs.

Chest expansion:

* Stand tall, legs slightly turned out from hips, feet hip distance apart.
* Hold hoop in front of chest; raise above head.
* Keeping torso long, let arms and hoop extend behind you as far as possible.
* Hold stretch for 30+ seconds.

Side extension:

* Bend right elbow toward right hip bone, stretching through left side. Hold.
* Repeat left side. Hold.

Hamstring stretch:

* With both hands on top of hoop, place hoop at arm's distance on floor.
* Let torso melt toward floor as you continue to stretch arms and lengthen hamstrings.
* Hold stretch 30+ seconds.

Torso twist:

* Step feet slightly wider than hips.
* Place right hand in the center of hoop and reach left hand to right ankle. Keeping hips square, roll hoop to left as you lengthen and twist.
* Hold stretch for 30+ seconds.
* Repeat opposite side.

Warrior stretch:

* Turn right foot to right and angle left foot slightly to right.
* Bend right knee into a lunge, knee over ankle.
* Reach to bottom of hoop with right hand, then extend right arm to ceiling as left arm bends and rests on hoop at left side.
* Hold stretch 30+ seconds.
* Repeat sequence.
* Repeat with left leg in lunge.

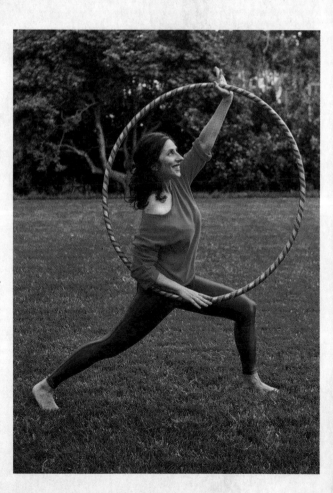

Tree pose

* Step feet together.
* Place both hands on top ⅓ of the hoop. Stretch arms overhead.
* Place one foot at ankle or inner thigh of opposite leg.
* Hold for 30+ seconds.
* Repeat opposite side.

Socializer Workout 2

Cardio workout 2: *The Jump Rope Combo—Med/High intensity Cardio*

If you're new to rope jumping, keep at it! It may feel awkward at first, but with time and practice, you'll get better and stay at it longer. In your first workout, you might jump only 30 seconds before switching to other cardio movements. Just build up when you're comfortable, and keep moving for 30 minutes. For higher intensity, increase interval time. Reduce interval time if you need to modify.

Props: Jump rope and flex band. Mat or soft surface.

Make sure rope is proper length for your height. Step one foot in center of rope; the handles should be approximately at your armpits. Lightweight plastic speed ropes are my favorite; they allow a much faster spinning rate.

Interval 1: Jumping Rope

Duration: 1–2 minutes

* Stand on level surface, knees soft, shoulders relaxed.
* Start by jumping with both feet. Then progress to "running" technique of alternating feet.

Interval 2: Knee-Ups

Duration: 1–2 minutes

* Hold rope; stand with feet parallel.
* Double up rope, bend elbows, and hold rope at waist height.
* Alternate lifting knees to meet rope.

Interval 3: Speed Skater

Duration: 1–2 minutes

* Hold doubled-up rope between hands.

- ★ Stand in first position: heels together, toes apart.
- ★ Lunge left leg back at slight diagonal toward right.
- ★ Simultaneously extend both arms above head, sweeping slightly to right.
- ★ Step left foot back to starting, pulling rope and left elbow toward left hip.
- ★ Repeat for 30–60 seconds per side.
- ★ Alternate lunges for higher intensity.

Interval 4: Sumo Squats

Duration: 1–2 minutes

- ★ Stand in wide plié position.
- ★ Double up rope and hold with both hands in front of chest, elbows bent.
- ★ Bend knees to squat while extending arms and rope overhead.
- ★ Add torso rotation for intensity.

High-intensity tips:

- ★ Increase the speed and duration of your jumping-rope interval. Add such techniques as double-unders and crisscross.
- ★ Engage shoulder and back muscles by pulling hands apart whenever rope is doubled in your hands.

Strength Training Workout 2: *Body Beautiful Combo*

Props: Mat or soft surface; flex band.

Sequence 1: Michelle Obama Arms!

Works deltoids, core.

Seated Arms

Part 1: Open and Close/Pull apart

- ★ Sit on mat in a C-curve position: pelvis tucked, rounded upper spine. Hold flex band with both hands shoulder height and distance.
- ★ Pull hands apart with control and light resistance.
- ★ Open band one inch farther.
- ★ Repeat 30 seconds.

Part 2: Lift and Lower

* Remain in previous setup.
* Keeping light tension, lift arms one inch above shoulders.
* Repeat 30 seconds.

Part 3: One of Each

* Remain in previous setup.
* Alternate Open and Close, Lift and Lower.
* Repeat 30 seconds.

Repeat above sequence 3x.

Sequence 2: Gorgeous Guns

Works lats, core, biceps, triceps, deltoids.

* Sit in C-curve position, legs extended.
* Place band around bottoms of feet.
* Bend your elbows to 90 degrees, keeping them at shoulder height.
* Poth hands toward shoulders.
* Repeat 30 seconds.
* Do single-arm pulls, 30 seconds each arm.
* Alternate arm pulls for 30 seconds.

Repeat sequence 3x.

Sequence 3: Posture Perfection.

Works posterior delts, lats, triceps, core.

* Sit with straight spine, legs extended. (If necessary, bend knees softly or sit on folded blanket.)
* Rotate thighs, heels together, toes apart.
* Place flex band around your feet.
* With straight arms and palms facing hips, pull the band back and behind.
* Repeat 30 seconds.
* Pull right arm 30 seconds; left arm 30 seconds.
* Alternate double-arm pulls with single-arm pulls for 30 seconds.
* For intensity, lift one leg.

Repeat sequence 3x.

Sequence 4: Core Crusher

Works core, quads.

* Continue to sit with straight spine, shoulders over hips.
* Wrap flex band around right foot. Left leg remains straight.
* Engage core; lift right leg several inches, using flex band as gentle assist.
* Hold 8 seconds.
* Repeat 3x.

Repeat sequence 3x.

Sequence 5: Hot Quads

Works core, quads.

* Sit in c-curve position.
* Place band around feet.
* Bend one knee toward chest. Then push away, keeping resistance strong.
* Repeat 8x.
* Switch legs.
* *Repeat 3x.*

Sequence 6: A Little off the Side

Works shoulder girdle, core, inner and outer thighs, glutes.

Part 1: Scissor Legs

* Tie knot in band and loop around each ankle.
* Lie on right side, supporting upper body with right hand and forearm. Don't collapse!
* Lift right leg to hip height.
* Repeat 8x.
* Switch legs.

Part 2: Turn-out

* Continue in same setup.
* Externally rotate leg so thigh faces ceiling.
* Lift leg toward ceiling.
* Repeat 8x.
* Switch legs.

Part 3: Turn-in

* Continue in same setup.
* Internally rotate leg so heel faces ceiling.
* Lift leg.
* Repeat 8x.
* Switch legs.

Repeat entire sequence 3x.

Flexibility workout 2: *The Flexibility Flow Combo (Beautiful Movement with Purpose)*

Props: Mat, jump rope.

Expand and flex

* Sit on mat with legs bent, feet on floor.
* Hold backs of thighs.
* Inhale. Lengthen spine as you expand chest.
* Exhale. Curl torso into a C-curve.
* Repeat 3x.

Articulate the spine.

* Lie on mat, keeping knees bent and feet on floor, arms long at your side.
* Tuck tailbone under and lift hips off the mat one vertebra at a time.
* Reverse movement.
* Repeat 3x.

Lengthen the legs

* Extend legs long on mat.
* Pull right knee into chest.
* Lengthen left leg with flexed foot.
* Hold 30 seconds.
* Switch legs.

Wring out the spine

* Lying on back, bring right knee into chest.
* Move arms to a T at shoulders.
* Roll right knee to left side of body, keeping shoulders connected to mat.

* Gently press right knee with left hand.
* Hold 30 seconds.
* Switch legs.

Stretch the hamstring
* Double up jump rope and loop around right foot.
* Keeping head, shoulders, and hips on mat; stretch right leg up to ceiling.
* Pull gently on rope to increase stretch.
* Hold 30 seconds.

Stretch inner thigh
* Maintain rope around right foot.
* With rope in right hand, lengthen right leg to right side.
* Hold 30 seconds.

Stretch outer thigh
* Maintain rope around right foot.
* Place rope in left hand.
* Draw straight right leg across body.
* Hold 30 seconds.

Open hips
* Return legs to center.
* Place both feet on rope.
* Bend knees; pull up to armpits.
* Put feet in air in "happy baby" position: knees over shoulders, ankles over knees.
* Pull the rope to increase stretch.
* Hold 30 seconds.

Fold over
* Place both feet on floor. Roll up to seated position.
* Make a wide diamond with your legs.
* Fold torso over thighs.
* Hold 30 seconds.

Stretch arms

* ★ Cross legs in front of you.
* ★ Interlace palms behind back. Use rope if needed.
* ★ Fold forward, lifting arms toward ceiling.
* ★ Hold 30 seconds.
* ★ Reach right arm across torso; use left hand to pull arm closer.
* ★ Hold 30 seconds.
* ★ Switch arms.
* ★ Hold 30 seconds.

Repeat entire sequence with opposite leg.

■■■

Supporter Personality Workout

I hear you, Supporter friends: you don't have time to mess around with workouts that don't work. So I've put together tried-and-true workout plans that you can easily shoehorn into your schedule. What's more, you can keep track of your progress as you go. You'll see yourself getting faster, stronger, and more flexible; if you're eating well, you'll be losing weight, too. Nothing motivates better than finding out that working out really *does* work!

Below you'll find workouts for cardio, strength, and flexibility. Your body needs all three, and ideally, three times a week. Combine weight training and flexibility, or cardio and weights, or all three of you can. They're quick, they're easy, and they're effective. Go for it!

Cardio Workout 1: *Elliptical Speed Intervals*

Prop: Elliptical machine with variable speeds and resistance.

Stick to the following time/resistance guidelines for a productive 16-minute session.

Minutes	Resistance	Intensity
0–3	3	warm up
3–5	5	medium
5–6	7	fast
6–8	5	medium
8–9	7	fast
9–10	9	fast
10–11	5	medium
11–12	7	fast
12–16	4	slow/cool down

Strength Workout 1: *Light-Weight Strength Building*

Props: Two hand weights, 2–3 lbs. each.

Sequence 1: The Roll Down
Strengthens posture, spinal flexibility, breath work.

* Stand tall, feet hip distance apart.
* Weights are in hands, arms at sides.
* Deep breath in, then exhale, keeping weight equal between heels and balls of the feet as you roll down into a forward fold.
* Softly bend knees while folded over.
* Exhale and roll back up to a tall standing position.
* Repeat 3x.

Sequence 2: Tricep Kickback
Strengthens core, post delts, lats, triceps.

* With weights in hands, slightly bend knees and hinge torso forward at slight angle.
* Lift straight arms back to brush your rib cage.
* With control, bend elbows fully, bringing weights forward, then extend back to straight line.
* Repeat 8x.
* Pulse 8x.

Sequence 3: The Push-away
Strengthens core, glutes, quads, delts, biceps, balance.

* Bend both elbows, bringing weights to shoulders, palms facing each other.
* Step right foot back into a lunge as you straighten arms and "push" weights away from your center.
* Step right leg back to center as you return arms to bent-elbow position.
* Repeat on right leg 8x.
* Repeat on left leg 8x.
* Alternate right and left leg 8x.

Sequence 4: Split Squat with Press

Strengthens core, glutes, hamstrings, biceps, deltoids, lats.

* From upright position, step back with right leg into a lunge. Bend both knees.
* With front left heel pressing down, lift right heel.
* Bend elbows shoulder height and distance apart, palms facing each other.
* As you lift hips slightly, press weights straight overhead, rotating palms away from each other.
* Lower hips and return weights to starting position.
* Repeat 8x.
* Switch legs, repeat 8x.

Sequence 5: Single-Leg Standing Row

Strengthens core, glutes, quads, hamstrings, rhomboids, delts, balance.

* Stand on right leg with left leg straight behind and lifted.
* With weights in hands, lower torso toward floor.
* Press both arms to floor; row weights to the chest, elbows open to the sides of the room.
* Repeat 8x.
* Switch leg, repeat 8x.

Sequence 6: Lateral Lunge

Strengthens core, pecs, delts, glutes, quads, hamstrings, balance.

* Stand tall, feet parallel and hip distance apart.
* Hold weights shoulder height and distance apart, palms up, arms straight with soft bend in the elbow.
* Step right foot open to a wide squat position as arms float open to a T.
* With straight back, lean forward slightly, dropping hips over heels.
* Step right foot back to starting position, stand upright, and bring arms again to shoulder distance apart.
* Repeat 8x.
* Switch legs and repeat 8x.
* Alternate legs 8x.

Flexibility Workout 1: *Yoga Sequence*

Prop: Yoga mat or soft surface.

Cat/Cow
* ⋆ Kneel on all fours for tabletop position.
* ⋆ Exhale; round spine up to the ceiling and tuck chin.
* ⋆ Inhale; drop belly, arch back, extend chest forward.
* ⋆ Repeat 3x.

Down Dog
* ⋆ From table-top position, tuck toes under and push hips to the ceiling.
* ⋆ Keep feet hip distance apart and wrists shoulder distance.
* ⋆ Bend knees deeply to let chest melt toward thighs.
* ⋆ Hold.
* ⋆ Press heels down to stretch back of legs.
* ⋆ Hold.
* ⋆ Alternate bending each knee 8x to stretch calves.

Twist
* ⋆ In Down Dog, place feet slightly wider than hips.
* ⋆ Bend knees deeply.
* ⋆ Place right hand in center of mat.
* ⋆ Reach left hand to outside of right ankle.
* ⋆ Spiral spine to the right while keeping hips level and forward.
* ⋆ Hold.
* ⋆ Switch sides and hold.

Forward Fold
* ⋆ In Down Dog, step feet toward the hands, bend arms, and hold on to opposite elbows.
* ⋆ Let head, shoulders and neck hang freely.
* ⋆ Hold.
* ⋆ Bend knees deeply and slide palms under feet, toes to wrist creases.

* Hold.
* Interlace hands behind back.
* Stretch knuckles up to ceiling.
* Hold.

Frog

* In folded position, step feet to edges of mat.
* Place hands between feet.
* Bend knees deeply, allowing them to open wide.
* Sitting your hips low, press palms together at your heart center.
* Hold.

Single leg split

* Bring hands back to mat in front of you, straighten legs, and move feet to parallel.
* With hands still on ground, extend the right leg back and toward the ceiling.
* Hold.
* Repeat opposite leg and hold.

Standing quad stretch

* Round spine up to a standing position.
* Balance on left leg. Bend right knee; lift right foot behind you.
* With right hand, reach for inside of your right ankle.
* Draw heel to glute as you stretch the quad and balance.
* Hold.
* Repeat other leg and hold.

Overhead stretch

* Stand with feet hip distance; stretch arms overhead.
* Let arms fall behind torso, keeping head and sternum lifted.
* Breathe deeply and expand chest, bending elbows open to sides of room.
* Hold.
* Return arms to your side and stand tall.
* Shrug shoulders to neck, then roll forward 3x and back 3x.

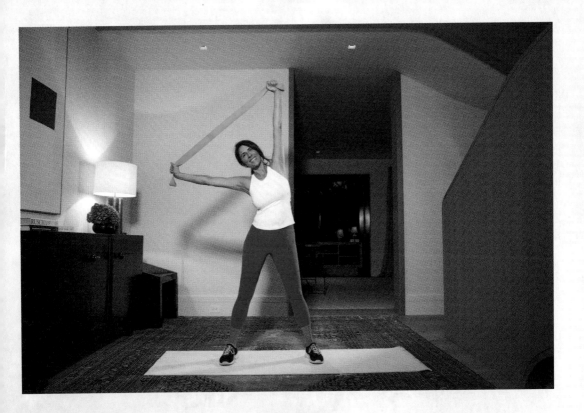

Cardio Workout 2: *Treadmill Speed Intervals*

Prop: Treadmill with variable speeds and inclines.

Duration: 30 minutes

Set treadmill incline to 1. Adjust times and speeds for a 30-minute medium/high-intensity cardio workout.

Minutes	Speed	Note
0–5	4	warm up
5–7	4.5	fast walk/jog
7–8	7	run
8–10	4.5	fast walk/jog
10–11	7	run
11–13	4.5	fast walk/jog
13–14	7	run
14–16	4.5	fast walk/jog
16–17	7	run
17–19	4.5	fast walk/jog + arm swings
19–20	7	run
20–22	4.5	fast walk/jog + arm swings
22–23	7	run
23–25	4.5	fast walk/jog + arm swings
25–30	4	cool down

Strength Workout 2: *Pilates*

Prop: Yoga mat or other soft surface.

Sequence 1: *Pre Roll-up*

Strengthens core, inner thighs; improves spine flexibility.

* Sit tall with knees bent, inner thighs and core zippered tight.
* Inhale. Exhale and lie back one vertebra at a time.
* Reach arms back in line with temples. Inhale.
* Exhale and sit up, with feet planted firmly on floor.
* Repeat 8x

Sequence 2: *Full Roll-up*

Strengthens core, inner thighs; improves spine flexibility.

* Sit with legs energized and stretched in front of you, shoulders over hips, spine straight.

* Inhale, lengthening through the crown of the head.
* Exhale as you tuck the pelvis and roll back onto mat, one vertebrae at a time.
* Reach arms back and in line with temples. Inhale.
* Exhale and sit up.
* Repeat 8x.

Sequence 3: Seated Balance C

Strengthens core, inner thighs.

* Sit in a C-curve position, pelvis tucked, upper abdominals curled.
* With bent knees and inner thighs firmly pressed together, place hands outside of ankles.
* Lean back slightly and float toes just off mat.
* Hold balance 10 seconds.

Sequence 4: Seated Balance T (tabletop)

Strengthens core, balance, inner thighs.

* Maintain same setup.
* Float shins higher into a tabletop position, parallel to floor.
* Move hands behind the thighs; float elbows open to the sides of the room.
* Hold balance 10 seconds.

Sequence 5: Seated Balance V

Strengthens core, balance, quads.

* Maintain same setup.
* Float shins higher into a V position.
* With legs straight and activated, move hands up legs toward ankles.
* Hold 10 seconds.
* *Pro tip:* Reset position if pelvis starts to wobble. Go back to seated balance C shape, then work back into the V form.
* For added challenge, extend arms in front of torso.

Sequence 6: Single Leg Pull

Strengthens core; improves breath work, precision, and control.

* Replace feet onto floor.
* Lie on back, pulling right knee into chest.

* Curl upper torso off floor.
* Float left leg off floor to the point where lower back wants to leave mat.
* With both hands on right ankle, exhale and pull right knee slightly closer to chest.
* Inhale as you switch legs.
* Repeat the exhale/knee to chest–inhale/switch legs sequence while maintaining C-curve position.
* Repeat 8 rounds.

Sequence 7: Double Leg Pull

Strengthens core; improves breath work, precision, and control.

* Maintain C-curve.
* Bend both knees into chest, heels touching, hands holding ankles.
* Inhale and extend arms and legs straight, inner thighs connected.
* Lower legs only to the point where lower back still connects to mat.
* Exhale, return to starting.
* Repeat 8x.

Sequence 8: Frog

Strengthens core; improves breath work, precision, and control.

* Maintain C-curve.
* Interlace the palms behind head with elbows wide.
* Keep heels together and toes apart, knees bent and slighter wider than hips.
* Inhale and extend legs straight.
* Exhale and bend knees back to starting position.
* Repeat 8x.

Sequence 9: Shoulder Bridge

Strengthens hamstrings, core, glutes.

* Replace feet and torso onto mat.
* Line feet up under knees, with inner thighs zipped.
* Tuck tailbone and peel your lower back off the mat into a shoulder bridge position.
* Bring left knee into chest; extend left leg to ceiling.
* Lift entire torso one inch, then return to starting.

* Repeat 8x slow.
* Repeat 8x pulse.
* Round down slowly, switch legs and repeat opposite leg.

Flexibility Workout 2: *Stretching*

Hamstring Stretch

* Lie on back with bent knees.
* Stretch right leg to the ceiling, hands around ankle, back rounding off mat.
* Hold 30 seconds.
* Switch legs.

Spinal Twist

* Still lying on mat, make a T with arms.
* With knees bent into chest and shoulders connected to the mat, let both knees fall to the right side of the body.
* Hold 30 seconds.
* Switch sides.

Ball

* On back, pull both knees into chest with arms wrapped around shins.
* Squeeze and hold 10 seconds.

Rolling

* Rock forward and back (only to shoulder blades) while holding ball shape.
* Massage muscles of spine while keeping core engaged.
* Repeat 8x.

Chest Expansion

* Roll to seated position, legs hip distance apart, toes pointed.
* Interlace arms behind back.
* Roll shoulders open while lengthening arms toward the hips and floor.
* Hold 30 seconds.

Saw

* Lie on back, arms in a T.
* Keep hips rooted to floor as you rotate upper torso to right.

* Reach left arm to outside of right ankle.
* Fold torso over right thigh and lengthen through fingertips, stretching arms away from each other.
* Hold 10 seconds.
* Switch sides.
* Repeat 8x.

Mermaid Stretch

* Sit tall with both legs bent to left side of body.
* Place right hand on mat, slightly away from right hip.
* Stretch left hand up and to the right. Keep arm in front of torso; hips remain rooted to the mat.
* Stretch left arm back up over head and lower to mat.
* Stretch right arm up and over to left.
* Repeat 4x.
* Switch legs to right side of body and repeat arm sweeps 4x.

■■■

Planner Personality Workout

Let's face it: the world needs more brains than brawn. But the world of exercise caters to brawn, not brains. That's why, my Planner friends, you've said "No, thanks" to boot camps, softball league, and Zumba classes. They are, in a word, shitty choices . . . for you. You thrive on analysis, perfection, strategy, and method. You like working independently. You like defined outcomes. Throwing a tire around with a bunch of grunters is just not your cup of tea.

So I've chosen workouts that maximize your strengths. You'll be working on your own with proven, measurable programs that improve cardio, strength, and flexibility. Make time for all three, three days a week, and you will not only lose weight, you'll become more focused and productive than ever. And you won't have to lift a single tire!

Cardio Workout 1: *Tabata Sequence*

This 16-minute workout features 32 30-second exercise sequences. You'll go through eight rounds of four different high-intensity moves; each round features 20 seconds of high-intensity work followed by 10 seconds of rest. (Sounds confusing, but it's really not.) No mat, no props. It's quick, efficient, and effective at getting your heart rate up and burning fat. Oh yeah, and it's fun!

Movement 1: Cardio Curtsy
* Stand with knees bent, abs engaged.
* Jump or step right, drawing left leg behind your torso.
* Extend right arm across body; reach it to floor with left arm lifted to side.
* Jump or step left, drawing right leg behind, and sweeping your left arm across.
* Repeat with dynamic pace 20 seconds.
* Rest 10 seconds.
* Repeat sequence 8x.

Movement 2: Cross-Body Mountain Climbers

* Start in plank position, shoulders over wrists.
* Bring right knee toward left side of torso, rotating hips.
* Alternate knees pulling toward chest.
* Repeat in dynamic pace 20 seconds.
* Rest 10 seconds.
* Repeat sequence 8x.

Movement 3: Plié Power-Up

* Stand in first position, heels together, toes apart, knees bent slightly open to sides of room.
* Keep torso upright, with arms low in front.
* Open arms and jump legs open to a wide plié.
* Power-jump both feet off floor and return to starting, arms closed.
* Repeat in dynamic pace 20 seconds.
* Rest 10 seconds.
* Repeat sequence 8x.

Movement 4: Low Squat (football "set")

* From plank position, pull abdominals in and up, slightly rounded in upper torso.
* Jump legs forward into a low squat, arms in front of chest.
* Return to plank position.
* Repeat in dynamic pace 20 seconds.
* Rest 10 seconds.
* Repeat the sequence 8x.

Strength Workout 1: *Light-Weight Strength Training*

Props: Light hand weights, 2–3 lbs. each.

Movement 1: Demi-Plié/Upright Row

Strengthens core, lats, delts, pecs, glutes, quads, inner thighs; improves posture.

* Holding weights, stand tall, shoulders over hips, heels together, toes apart.
* Press heads of weights together, palms down.
* Pull arms up, elbows out and leading, heads of weights pressed together.
* At same time, bend knees open to a demi-plié, heels together and firmly planted.
* Push arms down to starting position and stretch legs back to straight.
* Repeat 8x.
* Pulse 8x at top of movement.

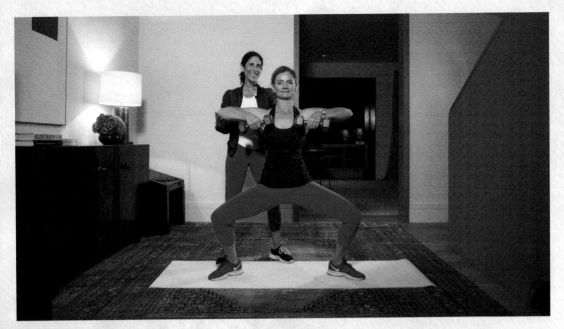

Movement 2: Demi-Plié/Delt Raise

Strengthens core, lats, delts, pecs, quads, glutes, inner thighs; improves posture.

* ✶ Remain standing, heels together, toes out, heads of weights pressed together, arms straight and lowered.
* ✶ Raise arms straight in front of you, bending knees open to a demi-plié.
* ✶ Lower arms and straighten legs.
* ✶ Repeat 8x.
* ✶ Pulse 8x with arms lifted.

Movement 3: Demi-Plié Relevé

Strengthens core, lats, delts, quads, glutes, inner thighs, calves; improves posture.

* ✶ With weights in hands, hold arms slightly wider than hips in front of torso.
* ✶ Lift heels high off floor (relevé position).
* ✶ Press heels together as you bend knees open to a demi-plié.
* ✶ Keep heels lifted as you bend and straighten legs fully.
* ✶ Repeat 8x.
* ✶ Pulse 8x, knees bent slightly.

Pro tip: For an added intensity and core challenge, repeat Movements 1 and 2 with bent knees and heels lifted (demi-plié relevé).

Movement 4: Hug a Tree

Strengthens core, lats, delts, pecs, quads, glutes, inner thighs; improves posture.

* Holding weights, palms facing each other, step feet open to wide plié.
* Lift arms to chest height, weights shoulder distance, elbows widened slightly.
* Open arms wide, then return to starting, keeping plié position.
* Repeat 8x.
* Pulse 8x with arms lifted out.

Movement 5: Arms to a T

Strengthens core, lats, delts, pecs, quads, glutes, inner thighs; improves posture.

* Hold plié from previous move.
* Open arms to a T: straight arms, palms up, shoulder height.
* Bring arms to front, shoulder distance.
* Return to starting position.
* Repeat 8x.
* Pulse 8x from wide T position.

Movement 6: Lift and Lower (Plié Hold)

Strengthens core, lats, delts, pecs, quads, glutes, inner thighs, calves; improves posture.

* Maintain plié position.
* Lift arms in front of torso, chest height.
* Lift heels to relevé position.
* Hold; return heels to floor.
* Repeat 8x.
* Pulse hips 8x from heel lift.

Alternate:

* Drop right heel; pulse 8x.
* Drop left heel; pulse 8x.

Pro tip: Add intensity by repeating Movements 4 and 5 in wide plié, heels lifted.

Flexibility Workout 1: *Full-Body Stretch*

Prop: Chair or table.

Forward Fold
* From arm's length distance, place hands on top of table or chair.
* With legs parallel and hip distance apart, softly bend knees, then melt torso toward floor.
* Hold.

Twist
* Keeping right hand atop table/chair, reach left hand toward right ankle, bending knees slightly.
* Slowly straighten right leg while maintaining ankle hold.
* Hold.
* Deepen twist by straightening both legs, hips drawing back evenly.
* Hold.
* Replace both hands on top of the surface.

Cat/Cow Stretch
* With palms on table/chair, exhale, tuck tailbone under, and round spine to ceiling (Cat stretch).
* Inhale and arch back, lifting torso slightly (Cow stretch).
* Repeat 4x.

Chest Expansion
* Interlace hands behind back, moving into forward fold.
* Let arms fall over torso toward table/chair.
* Hold.

Calf Stretch Lunge
* Using surface for balance, step right foot back into high lunge.
* Press heel to floor, stretching calf.
* Hold.

Hip Flexor Release
* Keep left knee in lunge; bend right knee with heel lifted.
* Lengthen and stretch the front of the right thigh (hip flexors).
* Hold.

Dancer
* ★ Using surface for light support, balance on left foot.
* ★ Reach right hand to inside of right ankle.
* ★ Press foot into the hand as you extend leg behind and up.
* ★ Hold.

Figure 4
* ★ Standing upright on left leg, place right foot over left thigh.
* ★ Keep torso lifted as you sit hips back.
* ★ Hold.
* ★ Sit lower; hold.

Repeat entire sequence using opposite leg.

Cardio Workout 2: *Treadmill*

Duration: 30 minutes

Prop: Treadmill with variable speed and incline.

Adjust treadmill speed and incline at time intervals below. Increase or decrease speed settings for higher or lower intensity, but maintain incline as recommended.

Minutes	Speed	Incline
0–2	3.5	3
4–6	3.5	5
6–8	4 walk	2
8–10	5 jog	1
10–12	4.2 fast walk	1
12–14	5.5 quick jog	1
14–16	4.2 fast walk	2
16–18	5.5 quick jog	2
18–20	4.2 fast walk	1
20–22	4 walk	2
22–23	6 run	1
23–23:30	6.5 sprint	1
23:30–25	5 jog	1
25–27	4.2 fast walk	3
27–30	3.5	2

Strength Workout 2: *Light-Weight Strength Training*

Prop: Light hand weights (2–3 lbs. each), mat.

Movement 1: Straight Arms—Lift and Lower

Strengthens core, lats, triceps.

* ⋆ Kneel on mat, knees hip distance apart, shoulders over hips.
* ⋆ Hold light weights, hands facing hips.
* ⋆ Hinge forward slightly, hips hovering just above heels.
* ⋆ Move straight arms back and out, reaching knuckles to heels.
* ⋆ Lift and lower arms one inch.
* ⋆ Repeat full range of motion 8x.
* ⋆ Pulse 8x.

Movement 2: Kick Backs

Strengthens core, lats, triceps.

* ⋆ Continue in kneeling position, hinged forward, arms long and back at sides.
* ⋆ Bend elbows, brushing ribcage and bringing weights forward, close to shoulders.
* ⋆ Repeat full range of motion 8x.
* ⋆ Pulse 8x.

Alternate:

* ⋆ Alternate one Lift and Lower with one Kick Back.
* ⋆ Repeat full range of motion 8x.
* ⋆ Pulse 8x.

Movement 3: Palms Up

Strengthens core, lats, triceps.

* ⋆ Continue in kneeling position, hinged forward, arms long and back.
* ⋆ Turn palms up to the ceiling and dust arms open to sides of the room.
* ⋆ Repeat full range of motion 8x.
* ⋆ Pulse 8x.

Movement 4: Circles

Strengthens core, lats, triceps.

* Continue in kneeling position, hinged forward, arms long and back, palms up.
* Draw circles, up, open, around and down.
* Repeat full range of motion 8x each direction.
* Repeat small range of motion 8x each direction.

Alternate:

* Alternate one Palms Up with one Circles.
* Repeat 8x circle one direction, full range of motion; 8x circle other direction, small range of motion.

Pro tip: If knees are sensitive, perform sequence standing with slight hinge at hip.

Movement 5: Lean Back

Strengthens core, glutes, thighs, delts, lats, pecs.

* Hold weights; kneel on mat, knees hip distance apart.
* Bring arms in front of torso.
* Lift arms slightly as you lean back.
* Hold position 4 breaths.
* Repeat 8x.

Movement 6: Side Kneeling Pendulum

Strengthens core, glutes, outer thighs, lats, shoulder girdle, delts.

* Hold weights; kneel on mat with knees hips distance apart.
* Tip entire torso to the right.
* Place right hand on mat directly under shoulder.
* Rest left hand holding weight on left hip.
* Extend left leg to left side of the room, lifting to hip height.
* Keep leg parallel as you sweep to front of the torso, then behind.
* Make range of motion large as possible while keeping torso perfectly still.
* Repeat 8x.
* Repeat 8x with the left arm/weight extended forward.

Movement 7: Side Kneeling Karate Kicks

Strengthens core, glutes, outer thighs, lats, shoulder girdle, delts.

- ⋆ Continue same setup.
- ⋆ Place left hand holding weight on left hip.
- ⋆ Flex left foot.
- ⋆ Bend left knee toward chest, then press leg out straight.
- ⋆ Imagine your heel hitting a bull's-eye with each press.
- ⋆ Repeat 8x.
- ⋆ Pulse 8x with left arm/weight toward front of room.

Movement 8: Side Kneeling Toe Taps

Strengthens core, glutes, outer thighs, lats, shoulder girdle, delts.

- ⋆ Continue same setup.
- ⋆ Rest left hand holding weight on left hip.
- ⋆ Straighten left leg, pointing toes, extending long through ankle.
- ⋆ Externally rotate leg, lifting to hip height.
- ⋆ Tap toe to floor in front of torso.
- ⋆ Lift left leg as high as possible while keeping torso still.
- ⋆ Tap toe to floor behind you.
- ⋆ Repeat 8x.

Movement 9: Side Kneeling Circles

Strengthens core, glutes, outer thighs, lats, shoulder girdle, delts.

- ⋆ Continue with same setup.
- ⋆ Rest left hand holding weight on left hip.
- ⋆ Extend left leg to wall in front of you. Maintain externally rotated thigh.
- ⋆ Reach left arm long to left side of room, in line with spine.
- ⋆ Lift leg as high as possible while keeping torso still.
- ⋆ Draw small leg circles.
- ⋆ Repeat 8x each direction.

Repeat entire sequence on opposite side.

Pro tip: If wrists are sensitive, prop torso with knuckles or elbow.

Flexibility Workout 2: *Contract and Expand*

Prop: Mat or soft surface.

Low Lunge
* From standing position, step right leg forward into a low lunge.
* Place hands on floor on either side of right foot.
* Maintain knee over ankle.
* Drop left knee/thigh to floor.
* Hold.

Hip Opener
* From lunge position, move right foot slightly wider than torso.
* Place hands to the center as your right knee opens to the right.
* Hold.
* Lower torso as you rest forearms on floor.
* Hold.
* *Repeat with opposite leg.*

Pigeon
* Bend right knee to right edge of mat, shin parallel to top of mat, foot to the left.
* Rest torso on thigh while left leg extends behind you.
* Hold.

Eagle Wrap
* Stand on slightly bent right leg. Bring left leg up and over right leg.
* Bring arms to a T.
* Cross left arm over the top of right arm; right arm under left.
* Overlap elbows; palms will meet in center.
* Hold.
* Draw crossed arms toward the ceiling as you inhale.
* Hold.

Eagle to Nest
* From Eagle position, round spine over thighs as you move elbows forward and away from center.
* Exhale and pull ribs back.
* Hold.

Chest Expansion

* From Eagle position, unwind arms, reach behind, and interlace fingers, palms trying to touch.
* Forward fold over thighs.
* Lift arms to ceiling.
* Hold.

Repeat entire sequence with opposite leg crossed on top.

Forward Fold

* Stand up; fold forward.
* Softly bend knees, reaching for the ankles, shins or floor.
* Hold.

Stand Tall

* Round up to standing, one vertebra at a time.
* Stretch arms over head.
* Reach right arm above left, to left side of room.
* Hold.
* Return to center.
* Reach left arm over right, to right side of the room.
* Hold.
* Return to center.

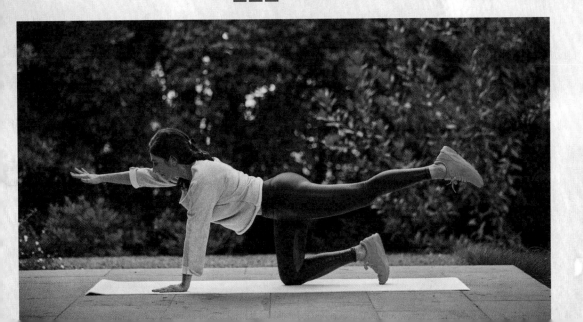

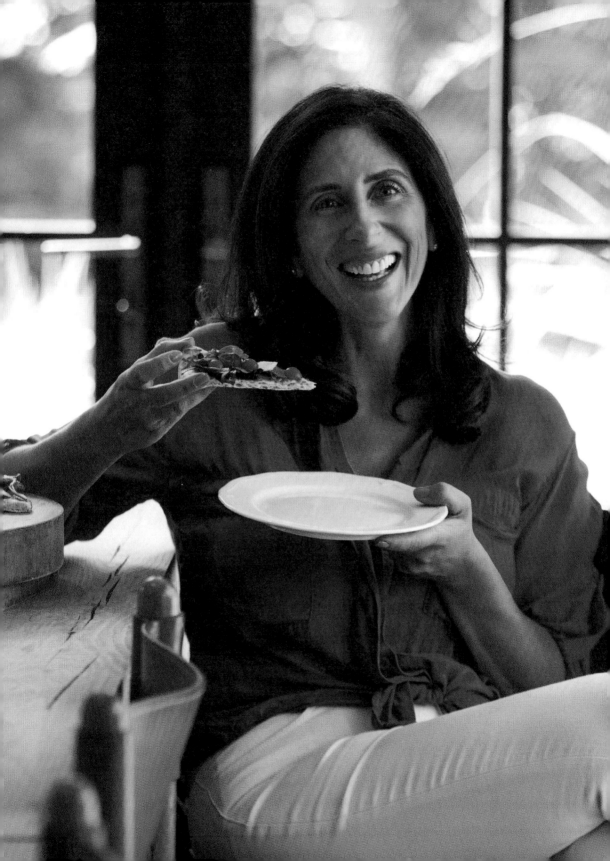

CHAPTER THIRTEEN

Your Favorite "F" Word: Food!

■■■

Eat It, Love It, Live With It.

QUICK QUIZ. WHICH OF THE following events in the movie *Wonder Woman* left our heroine with a look of unmatched ecstasy on her face?

a) Discovering that her wristbands deflect bullets

b) Roundhousing a bad guy in the moneymaker

c) Leading a heroic charge through No Man's Land

d) None of the above

Yes, fans, "d" is correct. WW's biggest smile resulted from wrapping those luscious lips around her first . . . ice cream cone.

And really, how unsurprising. In fact, the movie might have gotten an R rating if we'd seen WW tasting her first lobster claw or a ripe Chardonnay.

Sadly, though, we repeat dieters know that yummy food can be as double-edged as WW's Godkiller sword. (Just imagine that goddess physique of hers after 10 years on a Häagen Dazs® binge.) That's why so many of us feel we can't just "enjoy" food anymore. We're tired of figuring out diets, and the so-called diet "experts" out there are no help. *Drink skim milk! No, drink whole! Coffee is horrible! No, coffee is great, especially if you put butter in it!* (Who came up with *that* one?)

And while I'm at it, here's something else that deserves a rant: the word *diet*. Many of us hear it with the same enthusiasm as *slug trail* or *nail fungus*. And sure, I was one of them! *Diet* meant binge, forbid, and binge again. It meant abuse your body in the name of getting skinny. That messed me up in a *big* way.

But today I know this: dieting does not deserve a bad rap! The truth is, having a plan to lose weight is not only healthy, it's sometimes medically necessary.

So let's spend a minute reframing what "diet" really means.

1) *Diets are meant to be temporary.* Eating well is a lifetime pursuit, but actual dieting to lose weight is not a forever thing. So please don't freak out about never having a tasty morsel again. That's not how this works.

2) *Diets lead to sustainable change.* In real, nondieting life, there are no "bad" foods, no restrictions, no "cheat days." A true weight loss plan mimics real life in that you alter the portions and emphasize *modification* and *moderation.* Nothing is forbidden, and everything is adjustable!

3) *Diets are about quality and quantity.* You balance nutritious foods with portion control and . . . that's it! You lose weight.

4) *D-I-E-T: Delicious Intuitive Eating That lasts.*

And that's what this chapter is all about. This is your *Right Fit Formula* for food. You really *will* discover a way of eating that you can live with until death do you part. And I know, because I've spent years as a weight loss expert, working with thousands of people exactly like you. So when I tell you the following, I mean it. We're going to choose a way of eating in which you will:

1) Enjoy what you eat. For real.

2) Get to the weight that's right for you.

3) Be able to stick with it for life.

This chapter will break it all down and make it simple to plot your own unique course to eating well *for you.* No lectures, no one-size-fits-all/eat-this-or-be-damned menus. You know by now that the road to diet "failure" is paved with meals that someone forced you to eat. (*Boiled lettuce! It's good for you!*) Not here. You choose what works with your lifestyle, values, and body (and palate!), and I'll guide you every step of the way.

Why we eat what we eat

If I were to ask you, "What's the point of eating?" I'm sure you would give me one of the following sensible answers: "To fuel our bodies." "To give us energy." "To stay healthy." "To grow."

To which I would say, *yeah, right.*

For repeat dieters (Christine raises her hand), the point of eating has been anything *but* sensible. It's been all wrapped up with stress, emotions, wishes, fantasies, sadness, and just about anything *except* actual hunger. See if these scenarios ring a bell:

You're waiting for the cable guy. Boooorring.

You check out what's in the fridge. Open a couple cabinets. Ah. Forgot we had those Pop Tarts! Well, it's almost lunchtime.

You're waiting to hear about a promotion. When is she going to email you?

You poke around the kids' room. Those Butterfingers from Halloween—they don't go bad, right?

You didn't get the offer. Dang. You were perfect for that job! Why can't anything good ever happen to you?

You crack open the cabernet, call the pizza place, and throw yourself a nice pity party.

You just know they promoted that dingbat in Sales. He's about as qualified as a trained flea. Idiot. (Only you don't say "idiot.")

Where are those goddamn Butterfingers?

I think you get the point. And if you've come this far in the book, good news! You've already got lots of options for taking care of those feelings *without stuffing your face*. Which means we can start looking at some *easy* ways to eat for our best selves, not for our worst feelings.

Stepping off the diet roller coaster

More good news: we're about to reacquaint you with foods you enjoy. Yes, really. I know you've been conditioned to punish yourself with spray butter and fat-free mayo, but that nonsense stops here and now. This plan is all about working with *what is*—your likes, your lifestyle, your time and energy. You're going to choose *your* foods and learn to shop for them, prep them, and eat them in a way that will work for you and get you at your best weight. So let's get going!

STEP ONE: CHOOSE IT!

Yes, this step is pretty much as simple as it sounds. Just list the foods you like to eat and the foods you don't! Make a top 10 or top 15 list so that you can stick to the foods that really matter to you.

Don't be surprised if this feels a bit weird at first. If you've ridden the ol' Diet Merry-Go-Round a couple dozen times, you may have become completely disconnected to even knowing which food you enjoy! Writing it down will help you kick-start your feel-good relationship to food.

However, I do have a caveat. I want you to ground this list in reality. In other words, if your top five foods are mashed potatoes, steak, fried chicken, pizza, and ice cream, then you'd better be either a sumo wrestler or a farmhand. So when I say *choose food you like,* keep it to proteins, vegetables, fruits, and carbs.

Remember, the whole point is to build a healthy and sustainable relationship with food No one can sustain a healthy relationship with cheese-in-the-crust pizza. (And if Froot Loops or fried chicken really has to stay on the list, I'll show you how to deal with that later. We'll have choices that will satisfy your cravings without pushing you off your goals.)

Now, for each food on your "like" list, ask yourself these questions:

1) Does eating this food make me feel lousy, or good?

2) Is this food in line with my intentions and goals?

3) Do I enjoy eating this?

4) Does it taste good?

Food	Like	Dislike	Can't Live Without

You might want to stop and adjust your list at this point. If everything you listed tastes good but makes you feel lousy, try digging deeper for foods that you can embrace with a full heart and appetite.

5) *Is this food a Clog or a Cleanse?*

Cleanse foods are generally whole foods, such as fruits, vegetables, lean proteins, nuts, beans, and unprocessed grains. The *Clogs* generally include processed foods that are high in saturated fats and sugars: cookies, cakes, burgers, pizza, fries, pasta, foods in boxes and cans.

If you're still seeing a lot of food on your *Clog* list, fear not. We're not aiming for food sainthood, where you'll have to forego fatty favorites forever. We're aiming for awareness and balance. So hang in there, and we'll show you how to get there.

6) *Do the foods on my list balance one another? Do I consume relatively proportional amounts of fruits/vegetables, protein, carbohydrates, and fats?*

If you're like many people, your list might be light on the fruits and vegetables and heavy on everything else. So maybe you could stretch a little: without taking any favorites off the list, how about adding in some fruits and veggies? (Life, after all, is pretty boring with just corn, potatoes, and apples.)

Pro tip: Adding a fruit or veggie to each meal can significantly reduce the damage of unhealthier food choices. *And* you'll find it easier to maintain a healthy weight year-round.

7) *Do I generally buy these foods fresh, canned, or frozen?*

Fresh is always the best option, which is why I recommend shopping the outer aisles of the supermarket. Fresh-frozen is another good option for a whole food. And no, Tater Tots are not whole foods.

Pro tip: Keep frozen spinach, kale, or berries around for an easy go-to smoothie!

8) *Do these foods come in a box or can?*

Listen, I love macaroni and cheese, too. But boxed food is processed food, and processed food is something you want to keep to a minimum, or at least minimally processed. If you love crackers, for instance, pick whole grain. Choose Ezekiel for bread, which is made with sprouted grain. Find pastas made with whole grain or are gluten-free, or try making your own. I'll give you more options below.

STEP TWO: SHOP FOR IT!

Now take that favorite-food list and start shopping! Here's my recommended list of what to buy. When you stock your environment with high-quality foods, you can't help but make smart eating choices every time you open the fridge. As always, adjust to what works for you, and where possible, choose organic.

Proteins:

Lean steak, chicken and turkey, salmon, white fish

Pro tip: Grass-fed, hormone-free and wild-caught are the healthiest choices.

Low-fat Greek yogurt, cottage cheese, low-fat cheese

Pro tip: Go for low- or full-fat. Avoid fat-free, which has too many chemicals—and is also usually taste-free.

Beans: Kidney, chickpea, black beans, white beans, lentils

Milk: Low-fat, or almond or coconut

Hormone-free eggs

Fruits and veggies:

Blueberries, strawberries, raspberries (antioxidants, yo!)

Oranges (immune-system boosters)

Bananas

Spinach, broccoli, kale (dark greens are more nutrient-rich than light)

Sweet potatoes

Avocados (full of "good" fat, which removes plaque that causes heart disease)

Olive oil, coconut oil

Pro tip: To avoid pesticides, try to buy organic when choosing soft-skin fruits, like berries, peaches, plums, and grapes. Fruits and veggies with thicker skin, like bananas and oranges, are okay to buy nonorganic.

Grains:

Oats

High-fiber, minimally processed cereal

Brown rice

Quinoa

Whole-grain pasta

Snack foods and sweeteners:

Raw sugar

Coffee/tea

Low-fat frozen treats (these can stop you from hitting the Ben and Jerry's)

Whole-grain crackers (I like Van's Perfect 10, which are also gluten-free!)

Dried fruit: apricots, figs, prunes, raisins, cranberries

Nuts: Almonds, cashews, walnuts, pecans, pistachios (roasted and flavored). Packed with protein and manganese!

Seeds: Sunflower, sesame, whole or ground flaxseed.

Peanut butter (look for natural with no trans fats), almond or soy butter

Hummus

Dark chocolate

THE DIRTY DOZEN

According to *Good Housekeeping*, these babies get more than their share of pesticides. Some have traces of up to 60 different contaminants. Choose organic whenever buying fresh, or wash and peel what you can.

Apples

Celery

Sweet bell peppers

Tomatoes

Strawberries

Peaches

Nectarines

Kale

Grapes

Spinach

Cucumbers

Potatoes

THE CLEAN 15

These fruits and veggies generally carry a lesser share of pesticides. Organic is always great, but these guys get a clean bill of health either way.

Avocados

Cabbage

Mangos

Eggplant

Cauliflower

Sweet corn

Sweet peas

Papaya

Honeydews

Pineapples

Onions

Kiwis

Cantaloupes

Grapefruit

Asparagus

STEP THREE: STORE IT!

Back in Chapter 9 (Clean and Lean), you learned about my passion for glass containers, as well as my "divide and conquer" theory. As soon as I'm home from the grocery store, I divide all those veggies, fruits, snacks, and proteins into snack- and meal-sized units. Yes, it's a little bit more of a hassle than throwing the whole bag of whatever in the fridge. But the way I look at it, I'm helping out future Christine—the one who's going to be stressed, tired, and wanting food *now*. Future Christine, I'm well aware, would rather grab a bag of chips if the carrots aren't already cut up and ready to eat.

If you can relate, stock up on those glass containers! Throw your nuts and raisins together in single-serving snack bags; cut up carrots and celery and keep them crisp in a little water. The single-serving strategy is your best defense against overindulging. Divide and conquer, baby!

Pro tip: Divide your proteins (meat, fish, and chicken) into freezer bags after purchase. That way you won't need to defrost the whole package at one time.

STEP FOUR: PREP IT!

An equipped kitchen means you can ditch the preservative-laden, handy-dandy, so-called "convenience" foods. Grilling a chicken breast takes barely any more time or effort than heating up a Swanson's chemical cutlet. All that's needed is a little equipment and a can-do attitude. And boy, it's sure going to taste better.

So besides those glass containers and snack bags, you'll need the following kitchen supplies for preparing food that's easy and healthy:

Measuring:
Liquid measuring cup
Set of cups for solids
Set of spoons
A food scale (for those of you who like specificity!)

Prep:
Knives: Paring and carving
Cutting board (keep a separate one for meats and veggies)
Mixing bowls and spoons
Colanders

Grater
Vegetable peeler
Kitchen shears
Hand blender
Juicer
Food processor
Muddler (great for muddling fresh fruit into seltzer water for a quick, refreshing spritzer)

Cooking:

Saucepans: 1-, 2-, and 4-quart
Sauté pans: 9- and 12-inch
Baking sheet
Slotted spoons
Spatula
Tongs
Indoor cook-top griddle (great for grilling indoors)

Serving:

Small-plate dinnerware

Pro tip: Portion-control dinnerware is the secret weapon for keeping serving sizes realistic. *Slimware*, *For the chef*, and *Livliga* are some of my favorites.

Small cereal bowls
Custard bowls (great for servings of fruits and nuts)
Small mason jars
Small 4 oz. juice glasses
Coffee/tea mugs that inspire you! I love drinking from my bright yellow mug that says *Hello Beautiful*. Little things make a big difference.

On the go:

Thermal lunch bags
Small Tupperware for packable meals (Get tiny ones for condiments. No one likes a soggy salad!)
Ice packs to keep it cool
Ziploc bags: snack, sandwich, and quart size

Super Pro tip: Schedule it! Designate a weekly and daily time to prepare food. Scheduling ensures you'll stick to your intention to eat healthy portions.

STEP FIVE: PLATE IT!

When it comes to putting meals together, I have just three words: Balance, balance, balance. And I mean that literally: Three times a day, you're going to balance your intake of carbs, proteins, fats, fruits, and veggies.

Here's why. Different types of foods have different effects on your blood sugar. Blood sugar instability is the number-one physiological cause of a binge. After a sudden drop, you're starving, cranky, and must feed the beast *now*. That's not the best attitude to take to your refrigerator!

High glycemic foods, for example, are simple carbohydrates that break down in 30–60 minutes. They're fine for preworkouts, giving you that short burst of energy you need.

Examples: Nonfat yogurt, cereal, juices, smoothies, instant oatmeal, and yes, fruits (whole and dried).

Low glycemic foods are complex carbohydrates that break down in about 90 minutes to two hours. Because they're full of fiber, they keep you feeling fuller and will give you a little more bang for your blood-sugar buck.

Examples: Oats, rice, whole grain pasta/breads, sweet potatoes, and veggies.

Proteins take 3–4 hours to digest, depending on the protein. With protein, you sacrifice an energy rush but gain stabilized blood sugar. You also stay fuller and keep your metabolism active longer. That's exactly what you want. An inactive metabolism does *not* support weight loss, people!

Examples: Nuts, beans, lean meats, fish, poultry, eggs, milk.

Fats, meanwhile, can have a breakdown time from 6–8 hours. But in a healthy diet, your fat intake should be small enough not to affect your blood sugar and metabolism.

Examples: Oils, avocados, butter, cheese.

So the magic formula for energy *and* stability is to combine it all. If you bring together carbohydrates, protein, fats, fruits, and vegetables in each meal, you've got balance. Your blood sugar remains stable, and your metabolism works at its peak all day long. This staves off irrational hunger and supports a solid and satisfying meal plan. (Not to mention a slimmer waistline!)

To choose the right amounts for your metabolism and weight loss goals, keep reading.

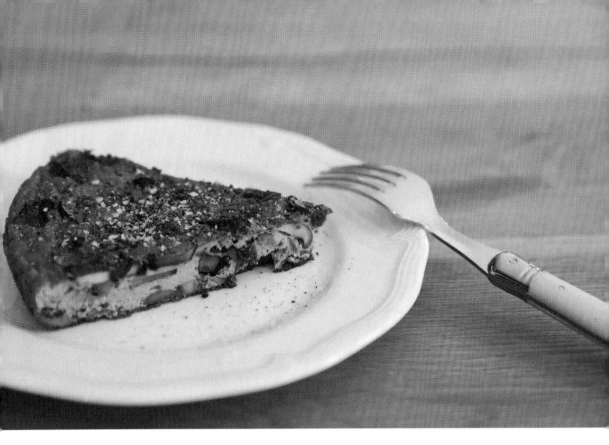

Plate Prepping 101

"Meat and two sides" seems to be a concept that's been around since cavemen days. (Mammoth steak with wild onions and a wheatgrass garnish? I can see that.) The fact is, it's not a bad concept! Combining protein with carbohydrates and fat gives both quick energy and a sustaining sense of fullness. But before you tuck into that caveman-approved burger and fries, let's check in with our 21st-century dietary needs.

What to eat:

Each person has different needs for carbs, protein, and fats. Athletes can tolerate (and need) more carbs and protein than nonathletes; active folks will need more calories than sedentary ones. Try the different combinations below, but honor your body's feedback. You might feel bloated with too many carbs, or too lethargic with too much protein.

If you are an average person maintaining good health and good weight,

What you eat is 40/30/30. That's 40 percent carbs, 30 percent protein, and 30 percent fat (with 10 percent or less saturated fat).

Your daily breakdown:

4 proteins—lean meat, fish, chicken, beans, nuts
5 fruits/vegetables
3–4 carbohydrates
3 fats

Your typical meals:

Breakfast: 1 protein, 1 carb, 1 fat, 2 fruits/veggies
Lunch: 1 protein, 1 carb, 1 fat, 1 fruit/veggie
Dinner: 2 proteins, 2 carbs, 2 fruits/veggies, 1 fat
Snacks: Protein/fruit

If you are an *active* person maintaining good weight,

What you eat is 55/25/20; 55 percent carbs, 25 percent protein, 20 percent fat. Most active people are able to consume more carbs without paying the weight price.

Your daily breakdown:

4 proteins
5 fruits/vegetables
5 carbohydrates
2 fats

Your typical meals:

Breakfast: 2 proteins, 2 carb, 2 fruits/veggies
Lunch: 2 proteins, 2 carbs, 2 fruits/veggies
Dinner: 1 protein, 1 carb, 1 fruit/veggie, 1 fat
Snack: protein, fruit/veggie

If you are **Christine,** your body and brain work a lot better on a high-protein diet, and carbs leave you feeling bloated and unsatisfied.

If you are you, pay attention to how your body operates best, and check the upcoming food plans for a lot more information about what to put on your plate.

How much to eat:

This gets interesting! It turns out that a serving of protein is *not* a Quarter-Pounder with Cheese or a Cracker Barrel buttermilk-fried half-chicken. WTF?!

Protein Servings

Meat: 3 ounces.
Dairy: ½ cup
Legumes: ½ cup

Fruits/Veggie servings

Leafy veggies: 1 cup
Fresh/frozen veggies: ½ cup
Fruit: ½ cup fresh; ¼ cup dried

Carb servings

Cereal: ½ cup
Rice/pasta: ½ cup cooked
Bread: 1 slice

Fat servings

Peanut butter, cheese, etc.: 1 ounce (spoonful of peanut butter)

Final thought: **Eating well is all about *quality* and *quantity*.** If you keep your food whole and fresh and your quantities reasonable, you're golden.

Use the charts on pages 224–225 to stay golden with your serving sizes.

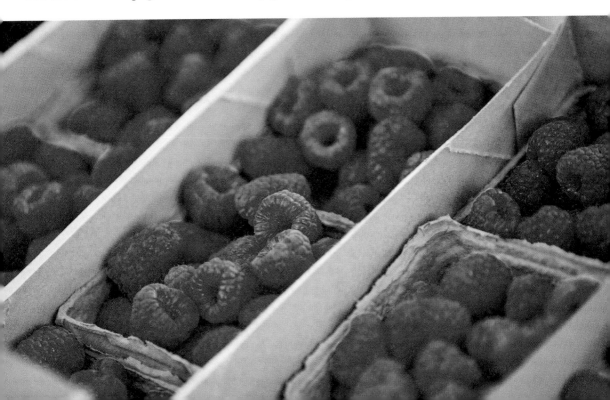

When to eat:

That's up to you and your lifestyle. Some people like to front-load their protein at break-fast and eat carbohydrates in the evening because that's what their body craves. Some like to dole it all out evenly throughout the day. Those who go hard-core with morning workouts like to carb-load early. Some folks like three larger meals per day; others prefer six small ones. (See the following chapter to see where you fit in.)

And the starring role on the plate goes to:

Well, it's not going to be fried chicken. No matter how you slice it, peeps, your healthy plate is usually going to be about half to two-thirds fruits and vegetables. (Simple math: the serving sizes are bigger, and there are more of them.) But you'll want to add protein and some grains in supporting roles to help you get the most out of each.

TIPS for staying the course:

* *Log it!* A monthly food log is a great way to stay connected to your choices. Log your daily meals for the first week of every month. Reevaluate and adjust as needed. Remember: flexibility leads to growth and rigidity to failure.
* *Pro tip:* Take photos of your food to check your actual portion sizes, use an app, or write out your food log. Lots of options for each personality!
* *Style it:* Let's face it: we're a society that celebrates the attractive. If you take a moment to make your plate pretty, you'll be much happier with eating it.
* *Hack it!* Eating well does not have to be complicated. If you're just not into mea-suring your proteins and carbs—or if you've eaten more than one meal this week over the kitchen sink—please turn the page. You'll get all my favorite tips and shortcuts for learning to intuitively pick the best foods for your lifestyle.

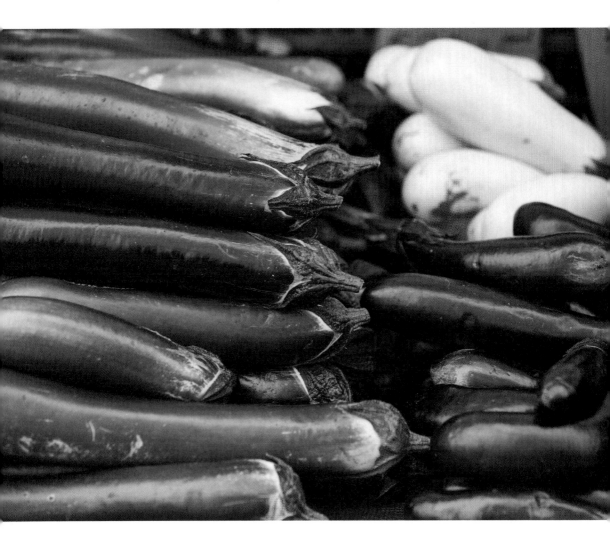

FRUITS + VEGETABLES

What counts as a serving?

FRUITS	VEGETABLES

FRUITS

ONE MEDIUM FRUIT

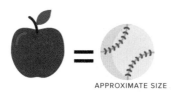

APPROXIMATE SIZE

FRESH, FROZEN OR CANNED FRUIT

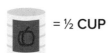 = ½ CUP

DRIED FRUIT

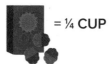 = ¼ CUP

FRUIT JUICE

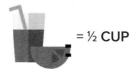 = ½ CUP

VEGETABLES

RAW LEAFY VEGETABLE

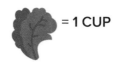 = 1 CUP

FRESH, FROZEN OR CANNED VEGETABLE

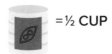 = ½ CUP

VEGETABLE JUICE

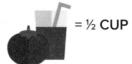 = ½ CUP

TRY FOR 4–5 SERVINGS A EACH PER DAY

Portion Size Guide

BASIC GUIDELINES

 1 CUP = BASEBALL

 1 TBSP = POKER CHIP

 ½ CUP = LIGHTBULB

 3 OZ CHICKEN OR MEAT = DECK OF CARDS

 1 OZ OR 2 TBSP = GOLF BALL

 3 OZ FISH = SMARTPHONE

 ## GRAINS

1 CUP OF CEREAL FLAKES = BASEBALL

1 PANCAKE = COMPACT DISC

½ CUP COOKED RICE = LIGHTBULB

½ CUP COOKED PASTA = LIGHTBULB

1 SLICE OF BREAD = CASSETTE TAPE

1 BAGEL = 6 OZ CAN OF TUNA

3 CUPS POPCORN = 3 BASEBALLS

 ## DAIRY & CHEESE

1 ½ OZ CHEESE = 3 STACKED DICE

1 CUP YOGURT = BASEBALL

½ CUP FROZEN YOGURT = LIGHTBULB

½ CUP ICE CREAM = LIGHTBULB

 ## FATS & OILS

1 TBSP BUTTER OR SPREAD = POKER CHIP

1 TBSP SALAD DRESSING = POKER CHIP

1 TBSP MAYONNAISE = POKER CHIP

1 TBSP OIL = POKER CHIP

 ## FRUITS & VEGETABLES

1 MEDIUM FRUIT = BASEBALL

½ CUP GRAPES = ABOUT 16 GRAPES

1 CUP STRAWBERRIES = ABOUT 12 BERRIES

1 CUP OF SALAD GREENS = BASEBALL

1 CUP CARROTS = ABOUT 12 BABY CARROTS

1 CUP COOKED VEGETABLES = BASEBALL

1 BAKED POTATO = COMPUTER MOUSE

 ## MEATS, FISH AND NUTS

3 OZ LEAN MEAT = DECK OF CARDS

3 OZ FISH = CHECKBOOK

3 OZ TOFU = DECK OF CARDS

2 TBSP PEANUT BUTTER = GOLF BALL

2 TBSP HUMMUS = GOLF BALL

¼ CUP ALMONDS = 23 ALMONDS

¼ CUP PISTACHIOS = 24 PISTACHIOS

 ## MIXED DISHES

1 HAMBURGER (NO BUN) = DECK OF CARDS

1 CUP FRIES = ABOUT 10 FRIES

4 OZ NACHOS = ABOUT 7 CHIPS

3 OZ MEATLOAF = DECK OF CARDS

1 CUP CHILI = BASEBALL

1 SUB SANDWICH = ABOUT 6 INCHES

1 BURRITO = ABOUT 6 INCHES

Power eating 101

TIPS AND HACKS FOR HAPPY TASTE BUDS AND A HEALTHY BODY

By now you know my mantra: Do what feels good. So for me, food not only has to be tasty and healthy, it has to be easy. And I mean drive-thru easy! If I can't instantly put my hands on something crunchy, yummy, salty, sweet—whatever I'm craving in the moment—then before I know it, I'm headed to an In-N-Out.

So now I'm laying it all out for you. Following are all the ideas I've gleaned from my 10,000 wrong diets (such as Apple Jacks for three months) and fifteen years of right ones. I've eaten it all, people, and I know what works! So take a look, soak it in, and dare yourself to start looking forward to driving past McDonald's a little more often!

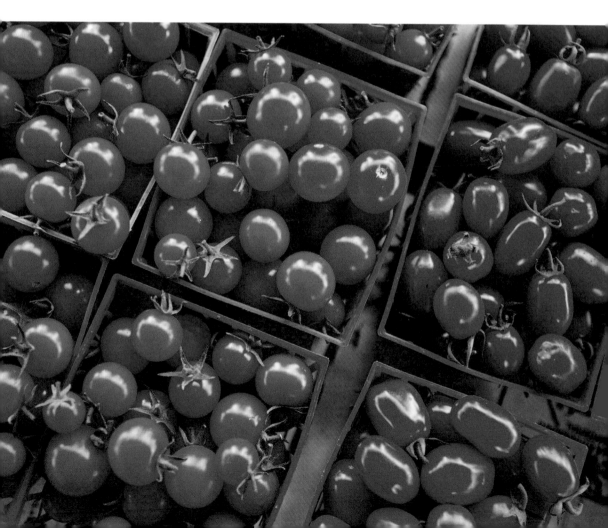

SUPERFOODS!
(OR, WHY POPEYE EATS SPINACH)

Whatever else you may eat today, add a few of these babies in your diet. Your body, and mirror, will thank you.

Super Berries!

Raspberry superpower: Fiber (20 percent per total weight), vitamin C, manganese, B vitamins, copper, iron, *and* antioxidants, which fight cancer-causing free radicals.

Pro tip: High-fiber foods are their own superpowers. They control blood-sugar levels, regulate bowel movements, require more chewing (which gives you time to register that you're no longer hungry), and make you feel fuller. High-fiber diets also tend to be less energy-dense, which means they have fewer calories for the same volume of food. Try lentils, artichokes, black beans, oats, and berries for high-fiber benefits. Hello, weight loss!

Strawberry superpower: Vitamin C (one serving equals 150 percent of daily value), fiber, manganese, folate, potassium, antioxidants.

Pro tip: Strawberries can carry a huge pesticide load, so purchase organic if you can.

Blueberry superpower: Antioxidant strength! Studies suggest they may reduce memory decline and heart-attack risk while providing other anti-aging benefits.

Blackberry superpower: Fiber, vitamins C and K, folate, manganese, and major antioxidants.

Cherry superpower: Vitamin C—nine times that found in a typical orange.

Pro tip: It's not available year-round, so look for supplements, juices, and powders.

Super Greens!

Spinach superpower: Fiber (double that of other greens), vitamins A and K, iron, folate and antioxidants.

Pro tip: Eat it raw in salads, or add a few handfuls to scrambled eggs, soup, pasta, or a smoothie.

Kale superpower: Vitamins A, C, and K; calcium; omega-3 acids; carotenoids (which protect eyes from UV rays); and fiber.

Broccoli superpower: Vitamins A, C, and K; folate; calcium; fiber; and cancer-fighting phytochemicals.

Brussels sprouts superpower: Vitamins A and C, folate, potassium, phytochemicals, and amino acids, which means high protein.

EAT THE RAINBOW!

Red foods contain Lycopene, an antioxidant known to maintain heart health. **Examples: strawberries, raspberries.**

Orange foods are rich in beta carotene and lutein, which help maintain healthy eye function. **Examples: carrots, pumpkins.**

Yellow foods contain fiber, iron, potassium, and folate, as well as other nutrients that help with the heart, skin, eyes, bones, digestion, and immune system. **Examples: Golden beets** (great for kidney health when juiced), **yellow dock** (eliminates toxins, improves blood health), and **dandelion** (helps with indigestion and weight control!).

Green foods are great sources of folate, which promotes healthy pregnancies and metabolizes amino acids for healthy cell division. **Examples: spinach, broccoli.**

Purple and blue foods contain antioxidants that help protect cells from damage and reduce risk of stroke, cancer, and heart disease. **Examples: blueberries, blackberries, eggplant.**

THE SWAP-IT SHOP

Looking for an upgrade from your fave form of junk food? Check out these offers:

You love: Flour tortillas
Swap for: Spinach, low carb, whole-wheat or corn options

You love: White bread
Swap for: Whole grain, sprouted, or Ezekiel

You love: Eggs in everything
Swap (at least some) for: Egg whites

You love: Baking with bleached white flour
Swap for: Baking with almond or sorghum flour

You love: Pancake syrup
Swap for: Pure maple syrup (go easy!)

You love: Waffles and pancakes
Swap for: Whole grain, gluten-free, or high-protein options (Vons and Traders Joe's have great ones)

You love: Baking with oil
Swap for: Applesauce

You love: Burgers and buns
Swap for: Turkey burgers on gluten-free or lettuce bun

Pro tip: Add chopped jalapeño, 1 tablespoon of soy sauce or teriyaki, and diced onion to ground turkey. Mix and grill. Yum!

You love: Fries
Swap for: Baked, sliced sweet potato. Drizzle with olive oil; add salt, pepper, paprika, and garlic.

You love: Pizza

Swap for: Homemade pizza! Use whole-wheat or gluten-free dough, add your fave grilled veggies, pizza sauce, and ¼ cup low-fat mozzarella cheese. The key is to manage your ingredients and portions.

Pro tip: If you're going out for pizza, eat one slice or order the salad or veggie pizza!

You love: Pasta

Swap for: Whole-wheat, spinach, or rice pasta

Pro tip: Believe it or not, a normal pasta serving is *very* small, about one-half cup cooked. *But* you can add your favorite veggies and protein to fill up your bowl. Here's one of my fave Italian staples: to a half-cup gluten-free pasta (I like everything fresh, including my pasta! I buy it in the refrigerated section), add broccolini and garlic sautéed in olive oil with a dash of sea salt. Then add either one slice of sausage or one 6 oz. piece of grilled chicken, diced. Sprinkle with a dash of grated cheese, and it's a well-balanced meal that includes carbs, proteins, and fats.

You love: Fried chicken

Swap for: A sautéed chicken cutlet breaded with panko bread crumbs or baked chicken breaded with cornflakes. Use white chicken breast and chop into smaller pieces.

Pro tip: A low-oil fryer requires only 1 tablespoon oil.

You love: Potato chips

Swap for: Wait for it . . . Regular fried potato or real veggie chips (the ones where you can see it was a veggie!). "Baked" chips or fake veggie chips have too many chemicals. Not healthy!

Pro tip: Make sure the vegetable is listed first in ingredients. Go for chips fried in sunflower or other good oil. I love North Fork potato chips. But don't eat the whole bag!

READ THE LABEL!

Nutrition Facts
Serving Size 3 oz. (85g)
Serving Per Container 2

Amount Per Serving

Calories 200	Calories from Fat 120

	% Daily Value*
Total Fat 15g	**20 %**
Saturated Fat 5g	**28 %**
Trans Fat 3g	
Cholesterol 30mg	**10 %**
Sodium 650mg	**28 %**
Total Carbohydrate 30g	**10 %**
Dietary Fiber 0g	**0 %**
Sugars 5g	
Protein 5g	

Vitamin A 5%	●	Vitamin C 2%
Calcium 15%	●	Iron 5%

*Percent Daily Values are based on a 2,000 calorie diet.
Your Daily Values may be higher or lower depending on
your calorie needs.

	Calories	2,000	2,500
Total Fat	Less than	65g	80g
Sat Fat	Less than	20g	25g
Cholesterol	Less than	300mg	300mg
Sodium	Less than	2,400mg	2,400mg
Total Carbonhydrate		300mg	375mg
Dietary Fiber		25g	30g

1) *Serving Size*

2) *Calories*

3) *Limit these*

4) *Get enough of these*

1) Here's a favorite: Clever food companies know a quick way to make their products automatically "healthier"—they increase the number of servings! Check that little bottle of strawberry smoothie: It doesn't look too caloric or sugary until you realize it's supposed to be two-and-a-half servings! Drink the whole thing, and you've ingested up to 600 calories and 60 grams of sugar. Buyer beware!

2) Whether it's cereal, nuts, bacon, trail mix—anything with a label—always multiply this number by the number of servings, just in case you're tempted to eat the whole darn thing.

3) For sodium and fat, you're going to want to keep this number at about 5 percent or less of recommended daily allowance. (That's about 120 milligrams sodium and 3 grams fat, including .5 grams saturated fat.) If you're looking at 20 percent or more (500 grams sodium and 15 grams fat), please back away slowly. That product is dangerous! Sugar, by the way, has no recommended allowance, so zero sugar is great! Otherwise, keep it under 5 or 6 grams.

4) We all love and need fiber and protein, but you don't have to go crazy. In fact, if you're eating lots of crunchy veggies, fibrous fruits, and whole grains, you're not going to need a lot of added fiber. And if you're making protein shakes *and* eating lean meats and chicken, you might be getting too much protein! That can be hard on your kidneys. A diet of whole foods is likely giving you all you need—fiber, protein, *and* necessary vitamins and minerals.

Ask these questions of your ingredient list:

* *Are there more than five ingredients?*
* *Do any of the ingredients exceed three syllables?*

If the answer to each is "no," you've got yourself a pass. Because:

* *The more ingredients, the more processing and preservatives required.*
* *The more unpronounceable the ingredient, the more likely your food product is a chemical stew of preservatives and artificial sweeteners. My favorite rule: When in doubt, go without!*

HEALTHIER OPTIONS
(TRUST ME: THEY STILL TASTE GOOD!)

If you like:

Refined sugar

Choose instead:

Honey, pure maple syrup, or sugar in the raw

Because:

Refined sugar raises your insulin level, which can depress your immune system, deplete your body of essential vitamins and nutrients, and promote storage of fat. Bottom line: a bigger bottom!! But don't go overboard on the honey and other natural sweeteners: sugar is still sugar, and your body will still experience that blood-sugar nosedive. Combine your sugar with fat, protein, or fiber to slow the absorption.

If you like:

Products with high-fructose corn syrup (check your fave soda, salad dressing, or nutrition bar)

Choose instead:

Products with natural sweeteners, such as honey or agave

Because:

The body processes corn syrup directly through the liver, then stores it as fat. Plus, you use up your body's vitamins and minerals processing those empty calories. *Bad idea! Do your best to avoid!*

If you like:

Products with bleached white flour

Choose instead:

Whole-grain or unbleached flour

Because:

The bleaching process robs flour of nutrients and fiber. Those empty calories will act on your body much as sugar does, spiking your blood sugar and setting off a craving for more.

If you like:
Products with artificial sweeteners, such as aspartame, saccharin, sucralose, and phenylalkaline (Check your fave cereals, pudding, popsicles, and low-fat yogurt)

Choose instead:
Natural sweeteners, like agave and sugar in the raw

Because:
These processed and unnatural derivatives of food and/or chemicals wreak havoc on your metabolism and energy levels and have been linked to cancer and Type 2 diabetes. These should be at the top of your *Not to Eat* list!

If you like:
Products with hydrogenated or partially hydrogenated oil

Choose instead:
Products with monounsaturated or polyunsaturated oils

Because:
Hydrogenated oils are trans fats. They have a higher melting point, which extends product shelf life, but at the cost of your arteries. You don't need the bad cholesterol (LDL) in your bloodstream! LDL is linked to coronary artery disease and cancer.

If you like:
Meat and dairy with saturated fats, such as butter, cream, hot dogs, and chicken skin

Choose instead:
Products that are high in heart-healthy Omega 3, such as almonds, olive oil, walnuts, sardines, avocados, and skinless meats.

Because:
Saturated fat can accumulate and clog arteries. Mono- or unsaturated fat actually acts as an arterial scrub-brush. It can clean your arteries of yucky plaque build-up. Plus it's got the same great "mouth feel" as saturated fat, which is the reason we love fats in the first place.

TAMING OF THE BUBBLY

Here's what we know about our favorite drinks: they taste good! They taste good because they have sugar (moonshine, frankly, isn't that tasty), and sugar sure helps the medicine go down. Plus they **feel** good, which leads to more alcohol, major snacking, poorly played pool games, loudly voiced opinions, and . . . more snacking.

Nevertheless, there are ways to fend off poor alcohol (and related) choices. My tips:

Go skinny. You can get light varieties of vodka, champagne, red wine, and beer.

Avoid the mixers. Use muddled fresh fruit and seltzer to dilute alcohol instead, and try a wine spritzer instead of straight wine.

Avoid frozen. Frozen daiquiris, margaritas, and piña coladas have way too many food additives and sugar. Plus you'll have to consume more to get the buzz you're looking for!

Water before wine! Always rotate in a glass of water for every glass of alcohol. Not only will you consume less alcohol, you'll stay hydrated for a proactive metabolism.

Drink slowly. Slowwwwwwly.

PSSSST! IF YOU READ NOTHING ELSE IN THIS BOOK, READ THIS!!

The tips below are what I call the *Right Fit* Foundation. Whatever your personality or lifestyle, these tips below are **essential** for making the most of your personalized weight loss plan. I feel so strongly about them that I promise this: if you follow these ideas, you will gain more energy and lose weight, *even if you do nothing else recommended in this book!*

So pay attention, yo!

Add a fruit or veggie to your plate. Every meal! And if possible, eat it before your meal. The fiber will take the edge off your craving, and the nutrition will balance whatever less-than-perfect choice you may be about to embark on. If you looooove Egg McMuffins for breakfast, for instance, I say go ahead and have one . . . but eat an apple first. (Better yet, eat two.) And if you notice a drop in your McMuffin consumption, well . . . you're welcome!

Always carry a snack and a drink! Our bodies often confuse thirst for hunger, so I never leave the house without a bottle of water in tow and some sort of snack (usually nuts and fruit). If I get too hungry, all willpower goes out the window. Savory satisfies me, so I always have hot onion garlic pistachios in my car. Put your top three satisfying snacks on your shopping list and keep them handy.

Eat your veggies; don't drink them. Yes, it's good to have cold pressed juices once in a while (4 to 8 ounces is fine), but it's a better habit to actually eat them. You get the full benefit of fiber and nutrients, not just the sugar!

Eat breakfast! Yes, it's really a meal not to be missed. You might think you're saving calories, but what you're really doing is blowing a hole in your metabolism. You get tired and lethargic, and then, guess what. *Bam!* Pizza for lunch! Work a healthy meal into your daily morning routine, at least before 10:00.

Stay hydrated! Use the pee test: if it's dark yellow, up your water intake! Try drinking a glass with every meal.

Pro tip: You can also hydrate with herbal teas or flavored water. (Make it yourself, please! The bottled stuff is full of chemicals). Watermelon and other fruits are also hydrating, with some nutrients and fiber, to boot.

Use supplements wisely. For many people, vitamins are largely useful for creating the richest pee in town. Your body can digest only so much! Unless your doctor tells you otherwise, you can get most of your nutrients just from eating whole food groups.

Pro tip: Trust your doctor for information on supplements. Not the pharmacist, not the Internet, not your know-it-all friend.

Swap out sweets and salts. Sweet-tooth people like me always keep fruits around the house. (I also love ricotta with honey as a dessert.) Nuts are great for salt-and-crunch lovers. The fiber and satisfaction can prevent a Doritos derail!

Eat without distraction. It's amazing how quickly food is consumed in front of a computer or TV. Don't grab it and shove it in your mouth. Put it on a plate, sit at the table, and mangia! Don't worry: your screen will wait for you.

Pro tip: Try a mindfulness exercise next time you eat. Think about how each part of your meal made it to the plate. Spend time chewing and savoring. You'll be more satisfied and grateful for the food you enjoy.

Prep, tidy, sit, eat. If you're a nibbler (hands up, Christine!), you tend to cook a little, eat a little. It adds up! So after you prep your food, make your plate and please put everything away. Then sit, eat, and enjoy.

Feed your workout. Fuel yourself with carbohydrates preworkout and consume protein after. Here's what I do. Preworkout, I fuel up with such carbs as yogurt, fruit, oatmeal, or toast with peanut butter. Postworkout, I eat eggs, nuts, or a meat-and-veggie bar. The essential amino acids in proteins build up the muscle that I just broke down. Plus, thanks to my now-stable blood sugar, I won't be craving a late-morning pig-out.

Sleep 6–8 hours. Lack of sleep inhibits good choices. (e.g., *I'm dragging. I can't work out today.*) It also inhibits leptin, the hormone that tells us when we've eaten enough. Don't believe me? Next time you sleep four hours, get back to me about your food choices and workouts that day.

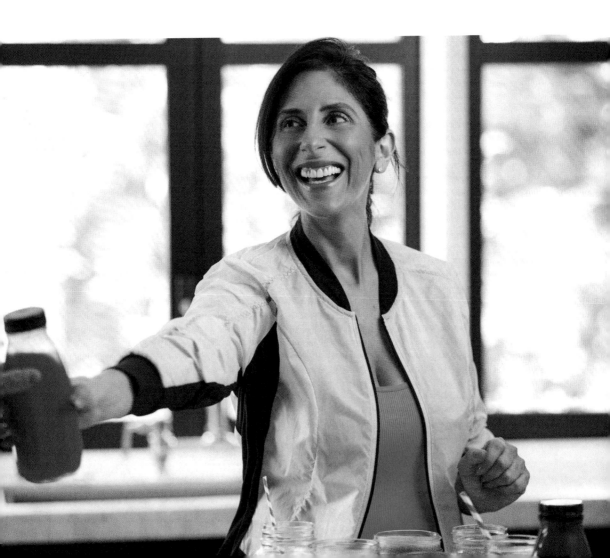

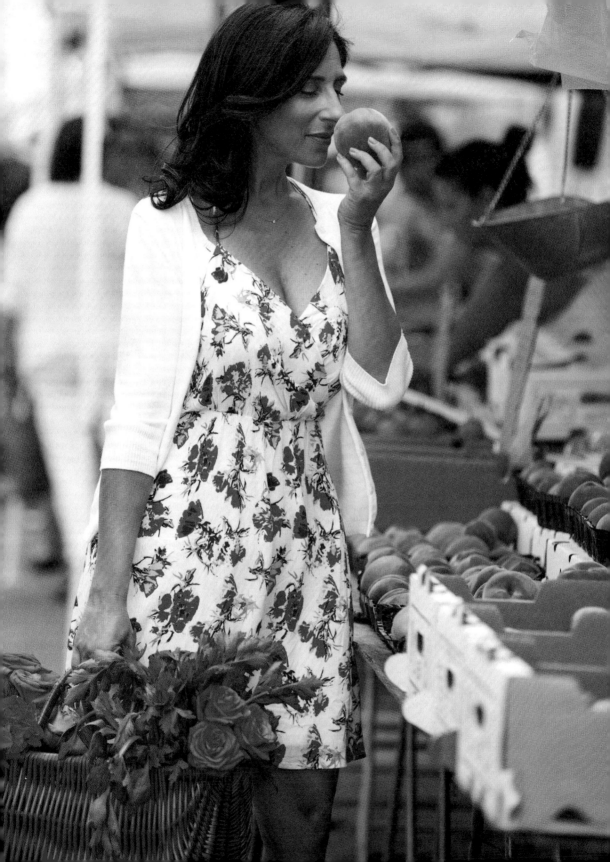

CHAPTER FOURTEEN

Step into the Fitting Room

Your Tailor-Made Weight Loss Plan

I'VE WORKED WITH MANY, many personalities over the past 15 years, and I can safely say they all have one thing in common: they want to lose weight. Other than that—nothing! We're all as different as our earlobes and fingerprints, so what works for Client Jim never seems to have the same effect on my Client Laura.

With that in mind, I can still say that you, dear reader, can find yourself in the following Weight Loss Profiles. By now you're fully aware of whether you're the take-charge Leader or the Supporter soccer mom with a houseful of responsibilities. So I've designed a program just for you that will capitalize on your strengths and keep you from slipping back into Yo-Yo Land.

The Leader Plan

Your food-choice profile: Streamlined. You need lots of quick, go-to options that will keep you from hitting the drive-thru.

Purchasing tips: Look for precut fruits and vegetables, ready-made salads with whole ingredients, single-serving trail mix or nuts, and ready-to-cook fresh veggies for stir-fry or kabobs. Make friends with the butcher and get your meats cut into the right-sized portions for your meals. Healthy meal kits, such as Blue Apron, are another great option for those on the go.

Cooking tips: Get to know your slow-cooker and your grill! You'll want easy, one-step meals.

Plating tips: Keep it clean. Fussy sauces and sides are not your thing.

Workout tips: Short increments (10–30 minutes) and high intensity work best for you. Get in, crush it, and get out! Just do it often enough to add up to three hours per week.

Stress-busters: Patience, grasshopper! Turn back to your stress chapter and practice getting more present with the body scan exercise or walking meditation. Do this daily.

Good idea to track: Your portions. Take photos of your plates for a week (we know you'll never write it down) and see if they're meeting your energy needs without going overboard. Do this weekly until you can get a good grasp on the quantity of your food. And track your workouts: Accomplishments fuel you! Bust out your Fitbit and keep an eye on what it tells you.

The Socializer Plan

Your food-choice profile: Creative. You'll want to try new recipes, share tips, check out ideas on Pinterest, and post food photos on social media.

Purchasing tips: Look for new, interesting, or seasonal items in the produce department and farmer's market. There's always a plethora of recipes that comes with the latest harvest of kohlrabi, pumpkin, or zucchini.

Cooking tips: You're a foodie, so prep and serving come naturally to you. Learn to modify your not-so-healthy favorite meals and to come up with innovative desserts that don't involve refined sugar or bleached flour. You've got the chops!

Plating tips: Make it pretty. Aim for color! It's so much easier to eat good-for-you when it *looks* good.

Workout tips: Join a group, any group! You'll love trying lots of different workouts as long as others are doing it, too. Most cities have as many workout options as coffee shops. Spin-yoga-Pilates-dance, anyone? I bet you would!

Stress-buster: Restoration. Because your favorite word is yes, which is *awesome,* you end up dashing all over the place. Check out a few of the grounding techniques that can help bring you back to the now and restore your energy for self-care.

Good idea to track: Your sensation of feeling full. Since you're pretty dialed into what you feel, use your strength to serve you. For the next week or two try checking in as you eat and stop at the first sign of fullness. It's likely you have a sweet tooth as well ("feeling" types often do), so try tracking sugar consumption, too.

The Supporter Plan

Your food-choice profile: Routine. You like to cook what you know how to cook, and to stick with what's good for you and your family. Your meals are like a Top 10 radio station: all hits, all the time!

Purchasing tips: Try working seasonal produce into your menu plans. And try exploring a few new places to buy food, like the farmer's market. Add a new recipe each week if you can.

Cooking tips: You're a pro at what you know, but try rotating some healthier choices into the regular menu plan. You can also try modifying family favorites that feature less-healthy ingredients. And nothing wrong with smaller portions of potatoes and bigger portions of broccoli! Don't forget to batch cook your food. You love to make enough for a few different meals.

Workout tips: Make sure it's a slam-dunk reliable workout. You don't want to mess around with gyms or workouts that don't fit your schedule. And put your workouts on the family calendar so everyone knows it's important.

Stress-buster: Notice your feelings. You're naturally a pretty cool customer, but you can be pushed to climb on the crazy wagon, too. The RAIN Practice on page 126 is perfect for your sense of logic and for working through what you feel in the moment. Practice weekly or as needed.

Good idea to track: Variety in your meals. Variety is satiety! Your default mode is the same ole same ole, but *beware*, this too has an expiration date. Rotating in new foods is an easy way to stay on target with your goals. And try doing an energy-and-body scan after your meals and workouts. You may be putting up with that chronic hip pain because you think it's supposed to be there. It's *not*.

The Planner Plan

Your food-choice profile: Thoughtful. You like knowing the rules around eating healthy food and you don't like to spend time experimenting. You like to *eat with purpose*.

Purchasing tips: Once you know what's best for your goals and lifestyle, shop for *only* those foods. If you need more vitamin C, for instance, put oranges, guava, and red peppers at the top of your grocery list. You'll maintain good eating habits without wrestling over what's in the fridge.

Cooking tips: Research the recipes that will work best with your time, food choices, and schedule. Have a go-to menu ready at the beginning of every week.

Workout tips: You like to know *why* you're doing a particular exercise, not just how. So have a trusted trainer work with you to create a workout blueprint. Schedule a regular time to make it happen.

Stress-buster: Letting go. You are my perfectionist friends, so remember that "done" is better than "perfect." Learn to let go of that which you can't control or what holds you back from being your best, and see Chapter 10 for tips. A daily practice would be ideal.

Good to track: Your nutrients. Good health is important to you, but you can lose track of what you're eating when you're caught up in work, worry, or frustrations. For the next week or two, take stock of how many whole foods you consume, and go back to your cleanse/clog log to help you out. Tracking your sleep might also benefit you in reaching your goals.

Your Menu, Your Way

I have a confession: Most diet plans trigger PTSD in me. When I read phrases like "¼ tsp. low-fat cream cheese" or "six baby carrots," I'm suddenly 20 years old again, freaking out because my mother bought low-fat milk instead of skim. Sorry, but I don't do rigidity anymore. Rigidity keeps me stuck in the land of Binge-Forbid-Binge, and I *know* it does for you, too! These days, freedom and choice are what keep me and *you* sane and healthy!

But I also know this: every one of my weight loss clients has said to me: *Tell me what to eat.* Plain and simple, they're afraid, and I can't blame them. When your default food choices come in Hamburger Helper boxes and McDonald's take-out bags, you're not the most confident planner of healthy menus. Not yet, anyway. So yes, I *can* tell you what to eat. I can help you plan menus—healthy weight loss menus—that will suit your tastes, lifestyle, and personality. Don't think of me as the Portion Police, ordering you to eat ⅛ of an avocado *or else.* Think of me as your Portion Cheerleader, urging on you lots of flexibility and choices for a healthy-eating lifestyle.

P.S. Some personality types prefer more guidance than others. Planners like their measuring cups, Leaders don't! So while each of my food plans is similar in nutrition, balance, and calories, they're all a little different in terms of options and portion suggestions. Find the one that is your Right Fit, and enjoy!

EMOTIONAL RESCUE!

Let's face it: A robot would be *great* at a weight loss program! After all, what drives ordinary mortals to consume TV, wine, and Cheetos? It's *feelings*, of course. So if a bout of anger, boredom, or anxiety is pushing you toward the Hershey bars, try these quick fixes to put you back on track.

The feeling: Boredom
Leads to: Mindless perusals through the cabinets and fridge.
Quick fix: Find a project! Write a thank-you note, have a "job jar," do a crossword. And if it's really bad, you have permission to play on your phone!

The feeling: Anxiety
Leads to: A hookup with the candy drawer.
Quick fix: Soothe it! Go for a half-hour run, take a hot bath, meditate.

The feeling: Depression/Sadness
Leads to: Secret eating, overeating, or bingeing.
Quick fix: If it's an ongoing mental health issue, get clarity. Seek a good therapist and work through it. If it's the ordinary blahs, put on some music and move through it. Go for a walk/run. Or watch what a friend of mine calls "mindless shit" for a half-hour—some silly YouTube videos or an old sitcom. (I'm addicted to reruns of *SATC* and *Friends*.) Just do it without the ice cream!

The feeling: Anger
Leads to: Impulsive eating. (Watch Bette Davis in *All About Eve* try to resist a jar of chocolates when she's fighting with her beau.)
Quick fix: A walk, a run, a bout of punching pillows, a venting session with your journal or your bestie, a gratitude list.

In short, you are not your feelings! Anger, anxiety, and boredom are just waves on the surface, and our strong, balanced selves are always waiting beneath. When we learn to value ourselves, we automatically begin steering away from self-soothing and taking healthy action instead.

The Leader Food Plan

Since I'm a Leader, too, I sympathize with you guys: You hate being told what to do, including what to eat! So I'm letting you take the lead in menu planning. (Which you would do anyway, but you know what I mean.) All you have to do is choose what looks good to you.

I know alpha types like food that's quick, easy, unfussy, and flavorful. That's why the drive-thru is so alluring: it hits all your sweet spots (although "flavorful" is debatable!). But guess what: a healthy menu can hit those sweet spots, too, *and* you'll have a lot more energy for running the world without an El Gordo Burrito sitting in your gut. So try out these healthy options . . .

Breakfast

If you like eggs:

Omelet made with feta, bell pepper, and spinach.

Fast options: Starbucks egg white/feta/spinach wrap; Au Bon Pain egg whites, cheddar & avocado on a skinny wheat bagel; Dunkin Donuts egg white flat bread

If you're on the move:

Smoothie made with Greek yogurt (about a half-cup), protein powder, frozen fruit, a little ice, and milk.

Even faster option: Starbucks peanut butter and banana smoothie.

If cereal is your thing:

High-fiber cereal with low-fat milk. Top with nuts and blueberries. Or add a small banana and nut butter (about a tablespoon) for your fruit and protein.

Granola (a few handfuls) on top of a cup of plain yogurt and fruit.

Oatmeal topped with nuts and yogurt (eat with a fruit, such as an apple), or topped with almonds and blueberries (add a hard-boiled egg for protein).

Pro tip: If you're a cereal dumper—half a box in the bowl—try portioning out your cereal into half-cup portions, or buy single-serving sizes.

If you like carbs:

Waffles (2 smallish ones) topped with blueberries and a small handful of shredded coconut. Have some milk and protein powder for balance.

Bagel topped with cream cheese (a spoonful or two), tomato, cucumber, and onion.

English muffin topped with almond butter and banana. Add a hard-boiled egg and some milk for protein.

If you like dairy:

Cottage cheese on a few crackers, topped with cinnamon and a little honey.

Fast option: Starbucks yogurt and fruit bowl.

Add-ons if you're still hungry (wait 15 minutes after eating):

Small apple with nut butter
Skinny latte
Kind bar
Handful of almonds or trail mix

Lunch

If you prefer salads:

Chicken Caesar made with romaine, sliced tomato (optional), shredded carrots, a handful of baked croutons, and about 3 ounces of diced chicken (about a handful). Toss with light Caesar dressing—but don't go crazy!

Chinese Chicken Salad made with fresh greens, red bell pepper, cucumber, peapods, and 3 ounces of diced chicken (about a handful). Top with a spoonful of slivered almonds and crunchy noodles, and dress lightly with Asian dressing.

Tuna made with 4 ounces of water-packed tuna (about half a can), mixed with a teaspoon of mayo, a teaspoon of honey mustard, and pickle relish. Serve with a handful of whole-grain crackers, a cup of veggie soup, and some carrots with hummus.

Fast option: Panera Bread modern Greek salad with quinoa.

For sandwich lovers:

Turkey Sandwich with 4 ounces sliced turkey breast (usually two slices) on whole-wheat bread with lettuce, tomato, and a few avocado slices. Honey mustard is a great low-cal condiment. Add an apple or fruit for balance.

Grilled Cheese Sandwich made with whole-grain bread and about 3 ounces of sliced cheese. Easy on the butter! Have a little minestrone, an orange, and a handful of almonds for a balanced meal.

Fast options: Starbucks smoked mozzarella and roasted red pepper sandwich; Chick-fil-A's grilled chicken nuggets

Pitas and wraps:

Apple and Cheddar Pita made with mustard, 3 tablespoons hummus, half a slice of cheddar cheese, mixed greens, and sliced tomato stuffed in a whole-wheat pita. Serve with apple slices.

BLT Wrap made with a tablespoon of hummus, a few avocado slices, a sliced hard-boiled egg, two slices turkey bacon, lettuce and tomato, stuffed into a whole-wheat wrap. Top with a little green goddess dressing and serve with grapes.

Salmon Wrap made with 4 ounces salmon, 2 tablespoons cream cheese, capers, red onion, and tomato in a warmed whole-wheat tortilla. Serve with an apple and baby carrots for balance.

If you're trying to resist that gut-busting burrito:

Bean and Cheese Burrito made with a handful of shredded Mexican cheese and a half-cup of black beans in a tortilla wrap. Warm until the cheese melts, and serve with salsa, leafy greens, and edamame with a little light dressing.

Faster option: Chipotle steak tacos with romaine, black beans, and fajita vegetables. Skip the sour cream; use fresh salsa instead.

Dinner

Break out the grill!

Grilled Steak (4–6 ounces sirloin) served with a small baked sweet potato, grilled asparagus, and a salad of greens and strawberries tossed with light dressing.

Grilled Chicken (6–8 ounces breast) served with quinoa, steamed broccoli, sliced pineapple, and a salad of leafy greens and mixed veggies, tossed with light dressing.

Grilled Salmon (4–5 ounces) served with a medium baked potato or yam, a tablespoon of sour cream (if you're using plain yogurt, feel free to use more), and a green salad tossed with light dressing.

The Perfect Burger (see page 264) served with watermelon and ¾ cup potato salad.

Grilled Fish (6 ounces mahi mahi) served with vegetables, leafy greens, and a whole grain roll.

Marinated Grilled Shrimp (see page 265) served with frozen mixed veggies sautéed in 2 teaspoons each soy sauce and sesame oil; a half-cup cooked risotto, and sliced mango.

Try out your slow cooker:
Shredded Pork and Beans (see page 264) served with cooked brown rice and several avocado slices.

If you're in the mood for comfort foods:
Baked Fish and Chips (see page 263) served with sweet potato fries.

Veggie Chili (see page 263) served with baked potato.

Layered Pasta made with 3–4 ounces ground beef or turkey sautéed with onions, bell pepper, a handful of mushrooms, and tomato sauce. Serve the meat mixture on ½ cup of cooked pasta. Serve with a Caesar salad made with romaine, a handful of baked croutons, and two teaspoons of Parmesan.

Stir Fry made with 10 ounces of tofu OR 4 ounces chicken breast and a few cups of mixed veggies. Stir-fry together in 2 teaspoons of peanut or sesame oil, adding 2–3 tablespoons stir-fry sauce. Serve with brown rice or wheat pasta.

Black Bean Quesadilla (see page 265).

If you're not in the mood to cook:
Greek Chicken Pasta Salad (see page 264).

Protein Smoothie Bowl made by blending a scoop of protein powder, a half-cup of low-fat milk, a half-cup of Greek yogurt, a cup of spinach and a small banana. Top it with strawberries, a handful of shredded coconut and a tablespoon of chia seeds.

Here's what a typical week's menu for a Leader might look like:

Leader	Breakfast	Lunch	Dinner
Monday	Feta/Spinach Omelet OR High-Fiber Cereal with Banana and Nut Butter (p. 246)	Turkey Sandwich OR Starbucks Chicken Artichoke Flatbread (p. 248)	Grilled Steak with Sweet Potato and Asparagus OR Baked Fish and Chips (p. 263)
Tuesday	Tomato Cucumber Bagel OR Granola 'n' Yogurt (p. 246)	Bean and Cheese Burrito OR Panera Greek Salad (p. 247)	Grilled Chicken with Quinoa and Broccoli OR Veggie Chili (p. 263)
Wednesday	Oatmeal with Nuts and Yogurt OR Starbucks Peanut Butter Smoothie (p. 246)	Chicken Caesar Salad OR Starbucks Mozzarella/Red Pepper Sandwich (p. 248)	Grilled Salmon with Baked Potato and Salad OR The Perfect Burger (p. 264)
Thursday	Chive Egg Scramble w/ Roasted Tomatoes OR Bran Cereal with Almonds and Blueberries (p. 246)	Chipotle Steak Tacos OR Tuna and Crackers with Veggie Soup (p. 247)	Chicken/Veggie Stir Fry OR Layered Pasta (p. 249)
Friday	Waffles with Coconut and Blueberries OR Starbucks Sausage/ Cheddar/Egg Breakfast Sandwich (p. 247)	Chinese Chicken Salad OR Turkey Burger Sliders (p. 270)	Grilled Fish with Veggies and Salad OR Slow Cooker Shredded Pork and Beans (p. 264)
Saturday	Oatmeal with Nuts and Blueberries OR Starbucks Fruit and Yogurt bowl (p. 247)	Healthy Tuna Sandwich OR BLT Wrap (p. 248)	Greek Chicken Pasta Salad OR Marinated Grilled Shrimp with Mixed Veggies and Risotto (p. 249)
Sunday	English Muffin with Banana and Almond Butter OR Starbucks Spinach/Feta/ Egg White Breakfast Wrap (p. 246)	Salmon Wrap OR Chicken Caesar Salad (p. 247)	Black Bean Quesadilla OR Pan Seared Soy-Glazed Salmon (p. 269)

See Glossary for more menu ideas and recipes.

The Socializer Food Plan

For you Socializers, eating is an art. You love food, you love fun, you love getting together with friends and trying new flavors and trends. That's why a meal of cottage cheese and baby carrots will send you straight to the pasta bar. Because you hate restrictions and rules (I'm with you) and you love pretty, I've cooked up options that will keep your body slim and your palate happy. And because you have just the teeniest tendency to nibble and overdo it, as most social people do, I'm giving you some portion guidelines and snacks. I also want to ask you to do three special favors for me. One: Please drink lots of water. That will keep you from putting something else in your mouth first. Two: Before you eat anything, ask yourself: *How hungry am I?* And three: Stop the instant you feel full.

Now, pick some favorites and have fun!

Breakfast

For sweet moods:

Peachy Oatmeal made with ½ cup cooked steel-cut oats, topped with a tablespoon of chopped walnuts, a little cinnamon, a teaspoon of chia seeds, and a cup of fresh or frozen peaches. Have a hard-boiled egg for protein balance.

Mango Rhubarb Smoothie made with a cup of 1% milk, ⅓ cup frozen rhubarb, ½ cup frozen mango, a tablespoon of shredded coconut, two teaspoons chia seeds, and ½ cup Greek vanilla yogurt. Blend with ice and ¼ teaspoon ground ginger. Yum.

Strawberry Nut Butter Waffle made with two small toasted waffles spread with a tablespoon of almond butter and topped with a cup of strawberries, ½ cup cottage cheese, and ¼ teaspoon cinnamon.

For savory moods:

Avocado Salmon Toast made with 3 ounces of smoked salmon and ¼ avocado spread on a slice of toasted rye. Serve with two clementines and ¼ cup low-fat yogurt.

Egg Sandwich made with a fried egg, tomato slice, chopped chives, and 2 teaspoons avocado mayo on a whole-wheat English muffin. Balance it with a couple dates for sweetness and fiber.

Power Protein Tortilla made with an ounce of melted low-fat shredded cheese on a whole-wheat tortilla. Top it with ⅓ cup cooked black beans and a fried egg; finish with salsa and cilantro.

For sweet-and-savory moods:

Ricotta Cinnamon Bagel made with 2 tablespoons low-fat ricotta and apple slices atop a toasted cinnamon half-bagel. Serve with one turkey sausage.

Sample Morning snack options:

- ★ Small apple with 1–2 tablespoons peanut butter
- ★ A granola bar and piece of fruit
- ★ Celery and a handful of wheat crackers with 3 tablespoons hummus
- ★ Orange and a half-ounce of almonds
- ★ Veggies & tzatziki sauce
- ★ A cup of Greek yogurt and a cup of sliced melon

Lunch

Tasty wraps:

Tuna Salad Lettuce Wrap (see page 273)

Turkey Feta Wrap made with 2 tablespoons hummus, ¼ cup diced roasted red peppers, 2 cups spinach, 2 ounces sliced turkey, an ounce of feta, and ¼ cup sliced cucumber in a whole-wheat tortilla.

Un-boring salads:

Chickpea Salad made with 1 cup rinsed chickpeas, 1 cup of spinach, and ½ cup grape tomatoes, topped with an ounce of feta and a teaspoon of light dressing.

Veggie Burger Salad made with a veggie burger patty cooked and crumbled over two cups of spinach, ½ cup chopped tomato, ½ cup cottage cheese, and ¼ avocado. Serve with watermelon.

Quinoa Salad with Edamame (see page 274)

Out-of-the-box options:

Baked Sweet Potato with Edamame (see page 273)

Protein Plate made with ½ cup sautéed Greek style lentils, and 3 scrambled egg whites. Serve alongside with a mozzarella stick and 1 orange.

Stuffed Avocado with corn salsa (see page 299)

Dinner

Southwest flavors:

Black Bean Zucchini Quesadilla made with ¼ cup rinsed black beans, ¼ cup cooked and diced zucchini, and 1 ounce cheddar cheese on a warmed tortilla. Fold in half and grill 1–2 minutes each side. Serve with salsa and a sweet kiwi for flavor balance.

Southwest Stuffed Avocado Shell (see page 273)

Big-flavor salads:

Quinoa Bean Salad (see page 275)

Chicken Kale Salad made with 3 ounces of diced chicken, 1 cup sliced strawberries, and two cups of kale, tossed with 1 tablespoon light dressing and served with a cup of lentil soup.

Easy palate-pleasers:

Whole-Wheat Pita Pizza (see page 274).

Stuffed Bell Pepper with Turkey (see page 275).

Tofu Sweet Potato Scramble (see page 274).

Sample PM Snack Options

* ★ Chocolate Hummus and strawberries (page 279)
* ★ ½ cup cottage cheese with pineapple
* ★ ½ cup low-fat ricotta with raspberries and honey
* ★ 3 ounces low-fat cheese with grapes
* ★ Grilled zucchini with blueberry salsa
* ★ 4 ounces warm milk with a dash of cinnamon (One of my faves)

Here's what a typical week's menu for a Socializer might look like:

Socializer	Breakfast	AM Snack	Lunch	Dinner	PM Snack
Monday	Peachy Oatmeal (p. 251)	1 small apple 1–3 tbsp. peanut butter (p. 252)	Tuna Salad Lettuce Wrap (p. 273)	Southwest Stuffed Avocado Shell (p. 273)	Chocolate Hummus (p. 279) ¼ c. strawberries
Tuesday	Avocado Salmon Toast (p. 251)	Mint Chocolate Smoothie (p. 284)	Baked Sweet Potato with Edamame (p. 273)	Whole Wheat Pita Pizza w/ Pineapple Mojito (p. 253)	½ c. cottage cheese ¼ c. pineapple (p. 253)
Wednesday	Pumpkin Smoothie Bowl (p. 285)	3 tbsp. hummus celery stalks 10 wheat crackers (p. 252)	Chickpea Salad (p. 252)	Black Bean Zucchini Quesadilla (p. 253)	½ c. low-fat ricotta ¼ c. raspberries drizzle of honey (p. 253)
Thursday	Ricotta Cinnamon Raisin Bagel with Turkey Sausage (p. 252)	1 orange 1 handful almonds (p. 252)	Summer Arugula and Mache Salad (p. 280)	Quinoa Bean Salad (p. 275)	¼ c. strawberries 1 oz. low-fat cheddar handful pretzels/nuts
Friday	Mango Rhubarb Smoothie (p. 251)	½ c. veggies and tzatziki sauce (p. 252)	Veggie Burger Salad (p. 252)	Stuffed Sweet Potato with Chorizo (p. 281)	½ c. Greek yogurt ¼ c. raspberries (p. 261)
Saturday	Power Protein Tortilla (p. 252)	2 small deviled eggs	Quinoa Salad with Edamame (p. 274)	Chicken Kale Salad with Vegetable Soup (p. 253)	4 oz. warm low-fat milk w/ dash of cinnamon (p. 253)
Sunday	Strawberry Nut Butter Waffle (p. 251)	1 c. Greek yogurt 1 c. sliced melon (p. 252)	Turkey Feta Wrap (p. 252)	Stuffed Bell Pepper with Turkey (p. 275)	Grilled Zucchini w/ Blueberry Chile Salsa (p. 253)

See Glossary for more menu ideas and recipes.

The Supporter Food Plan

You, my Supporter friends, are the backbone of every group and community, and your eating habits fit right in. You like foods that are tried-and-true, the kind you can create again and again and know you'll please any crowd. Who needs trends? The minute you see a line out a restaurant door, you beeline in the other direction. (*It's just food, people! Why would you wait an hour for $10 coffee and avocado toast, whatever that is?*)

But while everybody loves to gather around your dinner table, you do need some variety in your options if you're serious about losing those pounds. I'm not about to lay any razzle-dazzle on you, but I will shake up your routine just a tad, enough to jump-start a habit of healthier eating. Following are some easy ways to balance out your daily and weekly menus. Change can be good!

Breakfast

Instead of bacon and eggs, try:

Breakfast Burrito made with scrambled eggs (one egg plus two egg whites, scrambled with a teaspoon of olive oil and a tablespoon of water) plus ¾ ounce pepper jack cheese. Serve in a warm spinach tortilla with hot sauce. Add a cup of grapes for a fruit balance.

Open Face Tomato-Bacon Sandwich with 2 slices turkey bacon, 2 tablespoons avocado, 2 tomato slices, and a dash of crushed red pepper on wheat toast. Serve with a cup of vanilla yogurt and a small banana.

Instead of the usual oatmeal, try:

Oatmeal with Apple Butter and Walnuts, made with ¼ cup steel-cut oats cooked in 1 cup of 1% milk and mixed with a teaspoon of brown sugar and 3 tablespoons apple butter. Top with a tablespoon of chopped walnuts and serve with a hard-boiled egg for protein.

Instead of the usual yogurt and fruit, try:

Rye Toast with Yogurt and Pistachios, made with two slices of rye toast topped with 2 tablespoons each of ricotta, Greek vanilla yogurt, and roasted pistachios. Top with a drizzle of honey.

Strawberry Pistachio Yogurt Crunch, made with layers of Greek yogurt (one cup), sliced strawberries (¾ cup), and mini shredded-wheat cereal (⅓ cup). Top with a teaspoon of chia seeds and tablespoon of roasted pistachios.

Mango Peach Smoothie made with a blend of 1 cup 1% milk, ½ cup Greek yogurt, a cup each of frozen peaches and frozen mango, 2 teaspoons of chia seeds, and two scoops of protein powder.

Instead of an ordinary English muffin, try:

Apple-Peanut Butter Muffin with 2 tablespoons of peanut butter and ½ cup sliced apples served on a toasted whole-wheat English muffin. Serve with a ½ cup Greek yogurt topped with chia seeds.

Lunch

Instead of a burrito, try:

Bean Burrito Bowl made with romaine (1½ cups), cherry tomatoes (½ cup), rinsed black beans (1 cup), cooked brown rice (¾ cup), and chopped onion (2 tablespoons). Toss with a dressing of 2 teaspoons olive oil, ⅛ teaspoon cumin, and a tablespoon of lime juice. Top with a tablespoon of avocado.

Instead of plain chicken salad, try:

Caprese Chicken Salad made with 3 ounces diced chicken, ½ cup cherry tomatoes, and two cups of arugula. Toss with balsamic dressing (see page 289) and top with 4 mozzarella balls and crushed herb crackers.

Chickpea-Quinoa Fruit Salad made with ½ cup rinsed chickpeas, ¼ cup diced mango, and a cup of cooked quinoa. Dress with lemon vinaigrette (see page 289).

Instead of a burger, try:

BBQ Beef Salad made with corn (½ cup), romaine (2 cups), chopped tomato (½ cup), flank steak (4 ounces, cooked and sliced), rinsed black beans (½ cup), and chopped onion

(2 tablespoons). Toss with a dressing of 1 tablespoon light ranch and 1 tablespoon BBQ sauce. Top with 2 tablespoons tortilla strips.

Instead of the usual sandwich or wrap, try:

Greek Pita made with 3 ounces chopped chicken, ½ cup each cherry tomatoes and chopped cucumbers, and ¼ cup diced onion. Place in a whole-wheat pita and dress with 2 teaspoons wine vinaigrette. Top with a tablespoon of feta and a mint garnish.

Turkey Apple Brie Wrap made with two ounces of sliced brie melted on a spinach tortilla and layered with ½ cup apple slices, 4 ounces of turkey breast, and a cup of spinach.

Apple Cheddar Sandwich made with a slice of cheddar melted on two slices of sourdough, and filled with ¼ cup apple slices and 1 slice of prosciutto. Serve with a cup of blackberries.

Dinner

Instead of pizza or pasta, try:

Hawaiian Grilled Cheese (see page 289) served with a cup of tomato bisque.

Grilled Chicken Bruschetta (see page 290) served with roasted potatoes and a clementine.

Spinach Pesto Flatbread (see page 290) served with a cup of butternut squash soup.

Garlic Shrimp (see page 291) served with a cup of cooked linguini.

Instead of Taco Tuesday, try:

Mexican Turkey and Brown Rice Skillet (see page 291).

Instead of hot dogs or burgers, try:

Flank Steak with Watermelon Salad (see page 292).

Ginger Salmon (see page 291) served with a cup of cooked risotto.

Here's what a typical week's menu for a Supporter might look like:

Supporter	Breakfast	Lunch	Dinner
Monday	Open Face Tomato Bacon Sandwich (p. 255)	Red Beet Smoothie (p. 299)	Hawaiian Grilled Cheese (p. 289)
Tuesday	Simple Acai Smoothie Bowl (p. 293)	Caprese Chicken Salad (p. 256)	Grilled Chicken Bruschetta (p. 290)
Wednesday	Chooclate Protein Pancakes (p. 297)	BBQ Beef Salad (p. 256)	Salad Pizza (p. 304)
Thursday	Breakfast Burrito (p. 255)	Chickpea-Quinoa Fruit Salad (p. 256)	Grilled Garlic-Chili Shrimp (p. 294)
Friday	Apple Peanut Butter Muffin (p. 256)	Greek Pita (p. 257)	Mexican Turkey and Brown Rice Skillet (p. 291)
Saturday	Mango Peach Smoothie (p. 256)	Stuffed Avocado with Corn Salsa (p. 300)	Ginger Salmon (p. 291)
Sunday	Strawberry Pistachio Yogurt Crunch (p. 256)	Turkey Meatballs (p.294) with Zucchini Pasta	Flank Steak with Watermelon Salad (p. 292)

You'll find more recipes and menu ideas in the Glossary.

The Planner Food Plan

I love my Planner clients. They treat their bodies with 100 percent respect, and they do their homework when they're thinking about trying something different. Fads and trends? Forget it. They prefer experience, proof, and research. It might take some time, but once they're convinced that a diet or workout is going to work for them, they go all in.

So with that in mind, my Planner friends, I've crafted a food plan that meets your needs. Everything below is precisely portioned and proven for nutritional and weight loss value. And I've included snacks because we all know that the best thinking in the world can't defeat a rumbly, hungry tummy, so it's best to be prepared! You can create your own menus from the options below or follow the suggested menu plan. Remember to stock up on your healthy ingredients and ditch the items you know don't serve you. Enjoy the process of getting healthier!

Breakfast

If you normally go for cereal, try:

Coconut Porridge made with 3 tablespoons shredded coconut, 3 tablespoons almond flour, 1 teaspoon maple syrup, 1½ tablespoons flax meal, and a ½ teaspoon vanilla, all cooked for two minutes in saucepan containing ¾ cup almond milk.

Granola Blend made with a cup of almond or coconut milk blended with two scoops of protein powder and topped with ¼ cup granola and 2 tablespoons dried blueberries.

Yogurt and Granola Parfait made with a cup of raspberries, ¼ cup granola, and a cup of Greek yogurt layered in a glass. Top with a teaspoon of chia seeds and a mint leaf.

If you usually go for bagels or toast, try:

Veggie Bagel Sammy made with 2 tablespoons cream cheese, 6 cucumber slices, a small sliced tomato, and 2 slices prosciutto atop a whole-wheat toasted bagel. Top with sprouts.

Avocado and Beet Hummus Toast (see page 303).

Cinnamon French Toast (see page 306).

If you like eggs, try:

Sausage and Cheese Muffin made with a fried egg, a tablespoon of cream cheese, and a chicken-apple or turkey sausage link atop a toasted whole-wheat English muffin.

Morning Snack Options

* 1 ounce of crackers, 2 tablespoons hummus, and 5 dried apricots
* 3 dates and small handful roasted pistachios
* 2 tablespoons roasted chickpeas, 1 string cheese, and ½ cup red grapes
* Protein smoothie: 6 ounces rice milk, 1 scoop protein mix, ½ cup fruit
* 2 ounces fresh mozzarella w/ cherry tomatoes
* ½ cup cottage cheese, 6–8 bell pepper slices, 1 ounce (6–8) herb crackers
* Handful trail mix or ½ cup plantain chips + 1 apple

Lunch

Warm, balanced options:

Chicken Sausage, Kale, and White Bean Skillet made with 2 browned and sliced chicken-apple sausage links and 2 cups of kale sautéed in a tablespoon of olive oil with a teaspoon of minced garlic. Mix ½ cup rinsed white beans for a balanced meal of protein, carbs, and vegetables.

Sausage and Sauerkraut made with one browned and sliced chicken sausage link and ¼ cup sauerkraut added after browning. Serve with a cup of homemade or frozen roasted potatoes.

Salad option:

Wild Rice and Spinach Salad made by combining ⅓ ounce feta, 3 ounces chopped roasted turkey, a cup of cooked wild rice, and ½ cup soaked and drained sun-dried tomatoes. Place the mixture over 2 cups of spinach and dress with 2 tablespoons of balsamic vinaigrette.

Wraps and sandwich options:

Black Bean Avocado Wrap made with ½ cup rinsed black beans and ¼ avocado on a warmed spinach tortilla. Top with salsa.

Greek Flatbread made with 2 tablespoons hummus, 5 diced Kalamata olives, 1 ounce feta, ½ cup baby spinach, ¼ cup chopped tomatoes, and a tablespoon of chopped basil, all atop a toasted flatbread or pita.

Shredded Chicken Sandwich with ½ cup shredded chicken and ½ ounce shredded Monterey Jack cheese atop a toasted sandwich roll spread with 2 tablespoons light ranch dressing.

Chocolate Berry and Nut Butter Sandwich made with 1 tablespoon each of nut butter and chocolate-hazelnut spread on 2 toasted slices of sprouted grain bread. Top with cup mixed berries combined with ⅛ teaspoon lemon zest.

Dinner

Seafood Options:

Salmon with Avocado Salsa and Quinoa made with a mix of 2 tablespoons salsa verde, a tablespoon of cilantro, and ¼ avocado, placed atop 3 ounces grilled or seared salmon. Serve with ¾ cup cooked quinoa.

Sautéed Shrimp (see page 306) served with ½ cup couscous.

Meat options:

Beef and Broccoli (see page 306) served with ¾ cup cooked brown rice.

Cheese Tortellini with Ground Beef (see page 306).

Open Face Turkey Meatball Sub made with 2 tablespoons marinara sauce, 3 sliced turkey meatballs, and 2 tablespoons shredded Parmesan layered on half a whole-wheat hoagie roll. Bake at 400 degrees until cheese is melted.

Veggie options:

Mexican Stuffed Sweet Potato made by pouring 1 teaspoon coconut oil into a sliced baked sweet potato and topping with ½ cup corn, ⅓ cup rinsed black beans, 1 chopped scallion, 1 tablespoon cilantro, and salsa.

Candied Beet Salad made with 1 tablespoon candied pecans, ¾ cup cooked quinoa, ½ cup cooked beets, and 2 cups mixed greens, tossed with 2 tablespoons light dressing.

Afternoon Snack Options

* ⋆ ½ cup plain Greek yogurt and ¼ cup raspberries
* ⋆ ½ cup baby carrots with 2 tablespoons low-fat ranch, an ounce of jack cheese, and 3 Wasa crisps
* ⋆ 3 ounces lox and 6 Wasa crisps
* ⋆ 2 tablespoons hummus with 4–6 wheat crackers
* ⋆ 6 ounces chocolate soy milk and ½ ounce apple chips
* ⋆ 1 slice prosciutto, 3 crackers, and a ¼ of sliced apple
* ⋆ ½ cup plain Greek yogurt, with 2 tablespoons shredded coconut + ½ banana

Here's what a typical week's menu for a Planner might look like:

Planner	Breakfast	AM Snack	Lunch	Afternoon Snack	Dinner
Monday	Coconut Porridge	1 oz. crackers 2 tbsp. hummus 5 dried apricots	Chicken Sausage, Kale, and White Bean Skillet	½ c. Greek yogurt ¼ c. raspberries	Miso Crunch Bowl
Tuesday	Avocado and Beet Hummus Toast	3 dates small handful roasted pistachios	Black Bean Avocado Wrap	6 oz. chocolate soymilk ½ oz. apple chips	Salmon with Avocado Salsa and Quinoa
Wednesday	Veggie Bagel Sammy	1 serving roasted chickpeas 1 string cheese ½ c. red grapes	Greek Flat Bread w/ coconut spinach	½ c. baby carrots 2 tbsp. low-fat ranch 1 oz. jack cheese 3 Wasa crisps	Beef and Broccoli
Thursday	Orange Cantaloupe Smoothie (p. 307)	Protein Smoothie (p. 260)	Shredded Chicken Sandwich	3 oz. lox 6 Wasa crisps	Posole with Hominy
Friday	Yogurt and Granola Parfait	Caprese Salad (p. 315)	Sausage and Sauerkraut	2 tbsp. hummus 4–6 wheat crackers ¼ berries	Cheese Tortellini with Ground Beef
Saturday	Sausage and Cheese Muffin	¼ c. cottage cheese 6–8 bell pepper slices 1 serving herb crackers 1 orange	Wild Rice and Spinach Salad	½ c. Greek yogurt 2 tbsp. shredded coconut ½ banana	Candied Beet Salad
Sunday	Cinnamon French Toast	2 tbsp. trail mix ½ c. plantain chips ½ cup fruit in season	Chocolate Berry and Nut Butter Sandwich	1 slice prosciutto 3–4 crackers ¼ c. sliced apple	Sautéed Shrimp

You'll find more menu ideas and recipes in the Glossary.

Recipes for Each Personality Type

THE LEADER PROFILE

Big flavor, clean plate, convenient, easy prep

Baked Fish and Chips with Sweet Potato Fries

Serves 1

3 oz. white fish

1 egg white, beaten

¼ c. bread crumbs

¾ c. frozen sweet potato fries

½ tbsp. capers

¼ c. Greek yogurt

Parsley to taste

Lemon wedges

Preheat oven to 350°F. Clean and cut fish into 1-inch wide pieces. Dip in egg white and coat with bread crumbs. Place breaded fish pieces in oven-safe dish; bake 12–15 minutes until tender. Bake sweet potato fries according to package instructions.

Dipping sauce: Chop capers; combine with yogurt and parsley until mixed smooth.

Serve with lemon wedges.

Vegetarian Chili

Serves 1

1 medium baking potato

½ c. rinsed and drained black beans

½ c. rinsed and drained kidney beans

1 c. crushed tomatoes

½ c. zucchini, chopped

¼ c. corn

¼ c. onion, diced

1 tsp. ground cumin

1 tsp. chili powder

¼ c. low-fat Greek yogurt or light sour cream

Heat oven to 350°F. Pierce potato with fork and bake until soft, about 30–40 minutes. Combine beans, tomatoes, zucchini, corn, onion, and spices in saucepan; cook on medium heat, stirring, until heated through, about 15 minutes. Top chili and baked potato with Greek yogurt or sour cream.

The Perfect Burger

Serves 1

3 oz. ground beef patty

Lettuce

Tomato

Onion

2 tsp. mustard/ketchup

Small hamburger bun

Jalapeños, if desired

Grill patty to desired doneness and top with vegetables and condiments.

Slow Cooker Shredded Pork and Beans

Serves 6

1½ lb. pork tenderloin

1–15 oz. can black beans, rinsed and drained

1–24 oz. jar picante sauce

Combine pork, beans, and picante sauce in slow cooker. Cover and cook on low for 8 hours or until pork is tender. Shred pork and return to slow cooker for 10 minutes.

Greek Chicken Pasta Salad

Serves 1

½ c. cooked whole-wheat pasta

¼ c. rinsed and drained white beans

½ cucumber, sliced

3–5 Kalamata olives, pitted and sliced

¼ c. red onion, diced

3 oz. cooked chicken

1 oz. feta cheese

Dressing

½ tsp. dried or chopped fresh oregano

½ garlic clove, minced

2 tsp. lemon juice

2 tbsp. olive oil

Combine all salad ingredients. Whisk dressing ingredients, pour over salad, and gently toss to combine. Top with 1 oz. feta, crumbled.

Marinated Grilled Shrimp

Serves 6

3 cloves garlic, minced
⅓ c. olive oil
¼ c. tomato sauce
2 tbsp. red wine vinegar
2 tbsp. chopped fresh basil
½ tsp. salt
¼ tsp. cayenne pepper
2 lb. fresh shrimp, peeled and deveined
Skewers

In a large bowl, stir together garlic, olive oil, tomato sauce, and red wine vinegar. Season with basil, salt, and cayenne pepper. Add shrimp to bowl; stir until evenly coated. Cover and refrigerate 30 minutes.

Preheat grill to medium. Place shrimp on skewers. On lightly oiled grill, cook shrimp until opaque, 2–3 minutes per side.

Black Bean Quesadilla

Serves 1

3 oz. low-fat shredded cheese
2 tbsp. black beans
2 tbsp. corn
2 whole-wheat tortillas
1 tbsp. guacamole
¼ c. salsa

Heat a skillet or sandwich press. Combine cheese, beans, and corn in a bowl. Place mixture between two tortillas; heat on skillet or press until cheese is slightly melted or tortillas are golden brown, about 2 minutes per side. Serve with guacamole and salsa.

Citrus Herbed Grilled Chicken

Serves 4

1 tsp. fresh sage, finely chopped
1 tsp. fresh thyme, finely chopped
1 tsp. fresh rosemary, finely chopped
2 garlic cloves, finely minced
¼ c. extra-virgin olive oil
Zest of ½ lemon
2 tbsp. freshly squeezed lemon juice
½ tsp. natural kosher salt
4 boneless, skinless chicken breasts pounded to ¼ inch thick

Combine herbs, garlic, olive oil, lemon zest, lemon juice, and salt in large mixing bowl. Add chicken breasts and rub herb mixture all over. Cover bowl with plastic wrap and let chicken marinate for at least an hour, or overnight in the fridge.

Heat grill to medium. Grill chicken until cooked through, about 3–4 minutes each side.

Chive Egg Scramble with Roasted Tomatoes
Serves 2

4 large eggs (can substitute half for egg whites)
1 tbsp. unsalted butter
2 oz. Boursin garlic and herb cheese
1 tbsp. chives, finely chopped
Coarse sea salt to taste
Fresh cracked black pepper to taste

For tomatoes:

1 c. cherry tomatoes
1 tbsp. extra-virgin olive oil
1 tbsp. aged balsamic vinegar
⅛ tsp. coarse sea salt
⅛ tsp. fresh cracked black pepper

Beat the eggs together. Introduce lots of air for ultra-light, tender eggs. Season with pinch of salt.

Melt butter in skillet over medium-low heat. Add egg mixture. With spatula, push eggs across skillet in 3–4 motions. Repeat until eggs look slightly undercooked, about 2–4 minutes. Stir in cheese and chives and season with salt and pepper.

Preheat oven to 400 degrees. In medium bowl, toss tomatoes in extra-virgin olive oil, balsamic, salt, and pepper until evenly coated. Spread in baking pan and roast for 15–20 minutes.

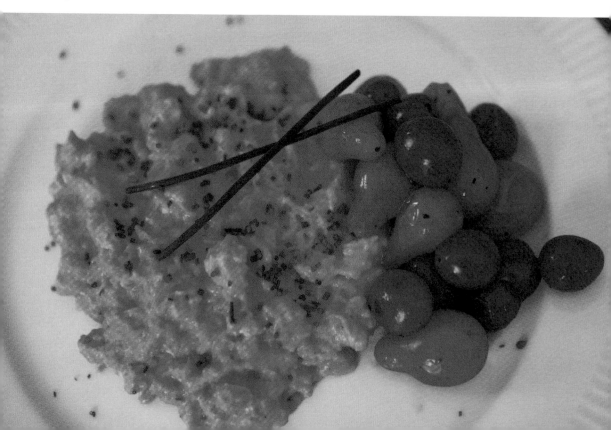

Healthy Tuna Sandwich

Serves 4

2 celery stalks, finely chopped

¼ small red onion, finely chopped

5-ounce can water-packed tuna, drained

¼ c. Veganaise® or lowfat mayo

2 tbsp. capers, drained, finely chopped

2 tbsp. fresh parsley, finely chopped

1 tsp. Dijon mustard

1 tbsp. fresh lemon juice, plus more if needed

Kosher salt

Freshly cracked black pepper

In medium bowl, combine celery, onion, tuna, Veganaise, capers, parsley, mustard, and lemon juice. Mix with until well combined. Season with salt, pepper, and more lemon juice, if desired.

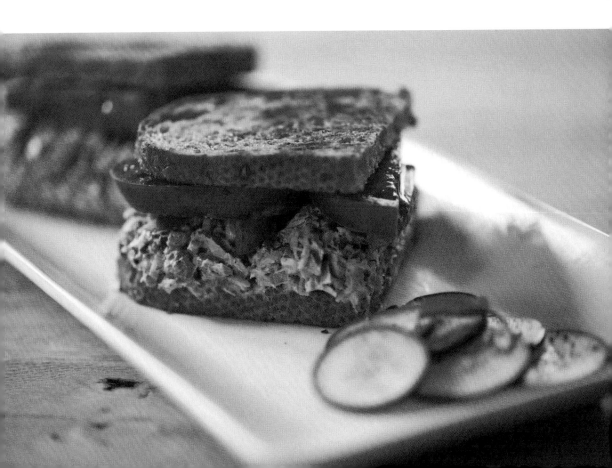

Healthy Teriyaki Grilled Chicken with Charred Broccolini and Brown Rice

Serves 4

For teriyaki sauce:

⅓ c. balsamic vinegar

⅓ c. raw honey

1 tsp. fresh ginger, grated

¼ tsp. freshly ground black pepper

1 tsp. miso

1 tsp. mirin (rice wine)

1 tbsp. water

For the chicken:

4 chicken breasts

Healthy teriyaki sauce

3 scallions, thinly sliced

⅓ c. fresh cilantro, roughly chopped

Roasted sesame seeds (optional)

Combine balsamic vinegar, honey, ginger, and pepper in small saucepan. Bring to a boil, lower to a simmer, and cook for 10 minutes. Add miso, mirin, and water, and let cool.

Marinate chicken in half of the sauce (reserve the rest) for at least 2 hours or overnight.

Heat grill pan over medium heat. Wipe off excess marinade and grill chicken 3–4 minutes per side, or until cooked through. Serve with remaining sauce and garnish with scallion, cilantro, and sesame seeds.

Charred Broccolini and Garlic:

Serves 4

2 tbsp. kosher salt

1 lb. broccolini (4 bunches)

3 tbsp. extra-virgin olive oil

4 garlic cloves, minced

Brown Rice:

Serves 6

1 c. short-grain brown rice

1 ¾ c. water

Kosher salt

In large pot, bring 8 cups of water and the salt to a boil. Remove and discard bottom third of broccolini stems. Cut any thick stems in half lengthwise. When the water boils, add broccolini, return to a boil, and cook over high for 2 minutes, until stalks are crisp-tender. Drain and immediately immerse broccolini in ice water to stop cooking. Drain and set aside.

Heat oil in a sauté pan. Add garlic and cook over low heat, stirring occasionally, for 1–2 minutes. Add broccolini and stir until heated through.

Rinse rice thoroughly until water runs clear. Place in pot with water and a big pinch of salt, over high heat. Bring mixture to a boil, lower heat, cover, and cook until all liquid is absorbed and the rice is cooked through, exactly 45 minutes. Turn off heat and let the sit for at least 5 minutes before fluffing it with a fork.

Pan-Seared Soy-Glazed Salmon

Serves 4

¼ c. reduced sodium tamari soy sauce (gluten free)

2 tbsp. raw honey

1 tbsp. unseasoned rice vinegar

1 tbsp. grated fresh ginger

1 tbsp. grated garlic

1 lb. wild salmon filet, cut into 4 pieces

1 ½ tsp. sesame oil

2 tbsp. scallions, finely chopped

In a large resealable plastic bag, combine soy sauce, honey, vinegar, ginger, and garlic. Add salmon pieces; toss to coat evenly. Marinate for at least 1 hour, or up to 8 hours, turning fish once. Remove salmon from bag, reserving marinade. Heat a large sauté pan over medium-high heat and add sesame oil. Rotate pan to coat bottom evenly, then add salmon. Brown for about 2 minutes, then flip and brown for 2 more. Reduce heat to low and pour in reserved marinade. Cover and cook until fish is cooked through, 4–5 minutes. Place salmon pieces on plate and garnish with scallions.

Sesame Soy Flank Steak Marinade

Serves 4–6

½ c. extra-virgin olive oil

1 cup tamari soy sauce

2 tbsp. sesame oil

3 cloves garlic, finely minced

2 tbsp. fresh peeled ginger, finely minced

1 tbsp. roasted sesame seeds

1 tbsp. coconut sugar

1 c. fresh cilantro, roughly chopped

⅓ c. fresh scallions, chopped

Zest and juice of 1 lime

Natural kosher salt

Fresh cracked black pepper

Combine all ingredients in a resealable plastic bag and shake until steaks are evenly coated. Marinate at least 4 hours or overnight. Season steaks with salt and pepper before grilling.

Turkey Sliders

Serves 4

20 oz. dark ground turkey or white for leaner taste

1 tbsp. Dijon mustard

3 tbsp. Worcestershire sauce

½ c. breadcrumbs

½ tsp. salt

2 c. diced caramelized onions, divided

6 mini brioche buns

1 avocado, chopped

4 medium tomatoes, sliced

6 oz. soft goat cheese

⅓ c. chives, diced

In a medium bowl, using your hands, combine turkey, Dijon, Worcestershire, bread crumbs, salt, and 1 c. diced caramelized onions. Form mixture into 3"–4" patties and place on a baking sheet. Refrigerate covered 1–2 hours. On a medium-high grill or skillet, coated with nonstick cooking spray, cook each burger for 2–3 minutes on each side. Meanwhile, toast buns to your liking. Assemble burger with avocado, a slice of tomato, a tbsp. of onions, a dollop of goat cheese, and a sprinkle of chives. Serve immediately.

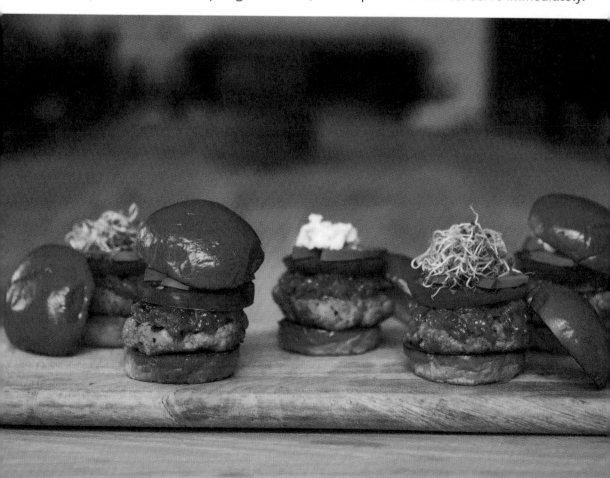

Coconut Bowl

Serves 1

1 young Thai coconut

½ c. vanilla Greek yogurt

½ c. diced mangos, raspberries, blackberries, and blueberries

½ tsp. coconut flakes

Crack open coconut. Drain water (save for drinking). Add yogurt into coconut, layer with fresh fruit, and top with coconut flakes. Best served chilled.

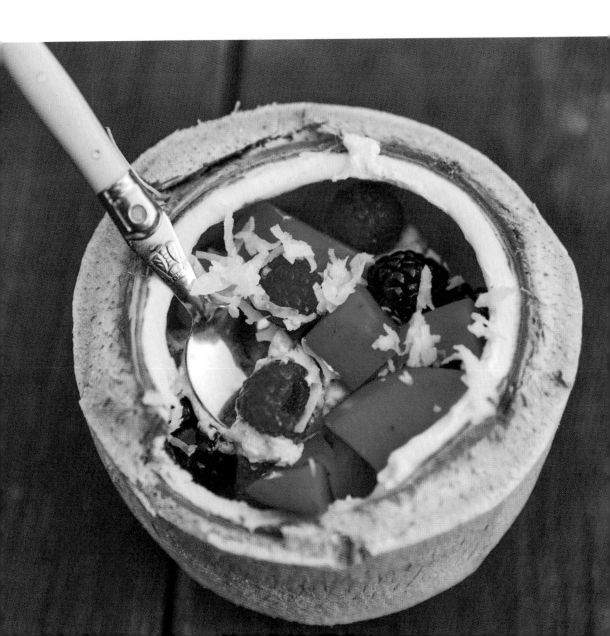

Baked Apples with Vanilla Ice Cream

Serves 6

½ c. raisins
¼ c. chopped pecans
¼ c. chopped walnuts
1 tsp. cinnamon
½ tsp. salt
3 tbsp. maple syrup
¼ c. brown sugar
6 apples, peeled, sliced, cored
Vanilla ice cream (optional)

Preheat oven to 350°F. Combine raisins, nuts, cinnamon, salt, and maple syrup in a large bowl. Mix in sliced apples and place in baking dish. Sprinkle brown sugar evenly on top. Bake until apples are soft, 30–40 minutes. Serve hot, warm, or room temperature with a scoop of ice cream.

Christine's Fave Sweet Snack

¼ c. part-skim ricotta
Dash of cinnamon and almond extract
½ banana, sliced
1 tsp. honey

Place ricotta in microwavable bowl. Stir in cinnamon and almond extract. Top with banana slices. Microwave 15 seconds. Top with a drizzle of honey.

THE SOCIALIZER PROFILE

Flavorful, creative, sweet-and-savory

Tuna Salad Lettuce Wrap

Serves 1

4 oz. tuna packed in water

3 tbsp. hummus

½ c. tomato, chopped

¼ c. celery, chopped

1 scallion, chopped

1 whole-wheat wrap

Lettuce leaves

Lemon juice, salt, pepper to taste

Mix tuna, hummus, tomatoes, celery, and scallion. Top wrap with lettuce and tuna mixture. Season to taste. Roll wrap and serve.

Southwest Stuffed Avocado Shell

Serves 1

½ avocado

½ c. rinsed and drained black beans

½ c. corn

½ c. tomato, diced

1 scallion, chopped

1 slice turkey bacon, chopped

Hot sauce to taste

1 tbsp. cilantro

Scoop avocado from shell; set aside shell. Combine avocado with beans, corn, tomato, scallion, turkey bacon, and hot sauce. Place mixture into shell and top with cilantro.

Baked Sweet Potato with Edamame

Serves 1

1 medium sweet potato with skin

1 tsp. coconut oil

1 tsp. chopped walnuts

Honey

½ c. shelled cooked edamame

Pierce potato with fork; place on a rimmed baking sheet lined in aluminum foil. Bake about 45 minutes, at 425°F until tender. Slit baked potato and top with coconut oil, chopped walnuts, and drizzled honey. Serve with edamame.

Whole-Wheat Pita Pizza
Serves 1

1 whole-wheat pita
1.5 oz. ground pork sausage
¼ c. mushrooms or bell peppers, diced
¼ c. tomato sauce
¼ c. shredded mozzarella

Toast pita in toaster oven/broiler for 3 minutes. Meanwhile, cook pork sausage, then sauté vegetables in pan. Spread tomato sauce over pita; top with sausage, veggies, and mozzarella. Place in toaster oven/broiler until cheese is melted.

Quinoa Salad with Edamame
Serves 1

½ c. cooked quinoa
½ c. cooked shelled edamame
¼ c. chopped cucumber
¼ c. chopped red onion
¼ c. chopped tomato
¼ c. grapes, halved
1 tbsp. chopped parsley
1 tbsp. chopped mint leaves
I tbsp. light dressing

Gently combine quinoa, edamame, cucumber, red onion, tomatoes, and grapes in small bowl. Top with parsley, mint, and dressing.

Tofu Sweet Potato Scramble
Serves 2

10 oz. extra-firm tofu
½ tsp. garlic powder
½ tsp. cumin
¼ tsp. chili powder
¼ c. thinly sliced red onion
½ c. chopped red bell pepper
½ tsp. sea salt
Pepper, to taste
2 c. spinach
1 c. baked sweet potato
Salsa
Cilantro, chopped
½ cinnamon bagel, toasted

Pat dry tofu. Wrap tofu in absorbent towel and press for 15 minutes with flat heavy object. Combine spices in small bowl and add enough water to liquefy. Sauté onion and pepper in 1–2 tbsp. olive oil until softened, about 5 minutes. Season with sea salt and pepper. Add spinach; cover to steam for 2 minutes. Unwrap tofu, crumble into pan with veggies, and sauté for 2 minutes. Add chopped sweet potato. Pour sauce over tofu; cook 5–7 minutes more until tofu is slightly brown. Serve with salsa, chopped cilantro, and toasted half bagel.

Quinoa Bean Salad

Serves 1

½ c. cooked quinoa

½ c. rinsed and drained white beans

½ c. steamed broccoli

½ c. chopped bell pepper

1 tbsp. light dressing

1 c. spinach

1½ tbsp. pine nuts

Combine quinoa, beans, broccoli, bell pepper, and dressing in bowl. Top spinach with mixture, then top salad with pine nuts.

Stuffed Bell Pepper with Turkey

Serves 2

2 medium green peppers

½ lb. ground turkey

3 tbsp. shredded cheese

1 tsp. chopped onion

¼ c. uncooked instant brown rice

½ tsp. Worcestershire sauce

½ tsp. salt

¼ tsp. pepper

1 large egg, beaten

8 oz. can tomato sauce

Heat oven to 350°F. Cut tops off peppers and discard. Remove seeds. Blanch peppers in boiling water for 5 minutes, drain, and rinse in cold water. In a bowl combine and mix well turkey, cheese, onion, rice, Worcestershire sauce, salt, pepper, egg, and half of tomato sauce. Stuff peppers with mixture. Place in ungreased baking dish. Pour remaining sauce over peppers, cover, and bake 45–60 minutes, until meat is brown and peppers are tender.

Creamy Chicken, Potato & Butternut Squash Soup

Serves 4

3 tbsp. olive oil

1 small onion, finely chopped

2 celery stalks, diced

1 medium carrot, diced

¾ c. butternut squash, cut into ¼-inch cubes

2 garlic cloves, crushed

2 medium potatoes cut into ½-inch cubes

1.5 lb. boneless, skinless chicken, cut into 1-inch cubes

3 c. of reduced-fat vegetable stock

1 bay leaf

1 6 oz. can cannellini beans, drained

1 c. spinach or escarole

2 c. low-fat milk

2 scallions, sliced

Sea salt & ground pepper to taste

2 tsp. cornstarch

Heat oil in large saucepan over medium heat. Add onion, celery, carrot, and butternut squash; cook 5-7 minutes or until the veggies begin to soften. Add garlic and cook until fragrant, stirring frequently, about 1 minute. Add diced potato, chicken, stock, and bay leaf; bring to slow boil over medium heat. Reduce heat and simmer 20–25 minutes, until potato and chicken are tender, stirring occasionally. Stir in cannellini beans, spinach, milk, and half the scallions. Cook 5 minutes or until heated through. Add salt and pepper to taste. Top with remaining scallions and serve. Note: To thicken soup, mix cornstarch with 2 tbsp. soup liquid. Add to pot and cook until soup thickens, about 2-3 minutes.

Healthy Soda

¼ c. fruit (pineapple, melons, berries, etc.)

10 oz. seltzer water

Muddle fruit in small cup. Pour fruit into seltzer water; add sprig of mint if desired. Yummy and good for you!

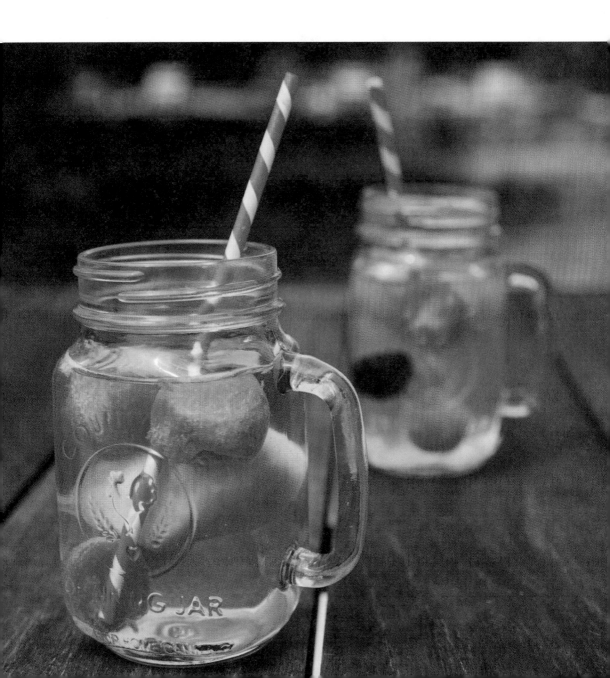

Pineapple Mojito

Serves 2

2 c. kale, stems removed
¼ c. fresh mint leaves
2 c. unsweetened coconut water
3 c. chopped pineapple
Juice of 1 lime

Blend kale, mint, and coconut water until smooth. Add pineapple and lime juice and blend again.

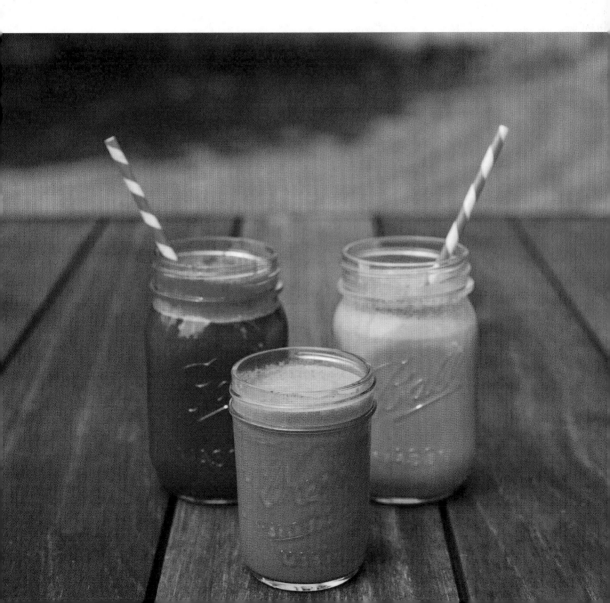

Chocolate Hummus

Serves 6

1½ c. or 1 15 oz. can no-salt black beans, drained

4 medjool dates, pitted

¼ c. raw almonds

¼ c. natural cocoa powder

1 tsp. alcohol-free vanilla extract

¼ tsp. cinnamon

¼ c. unsweetened almond milk

Blend all ingredients. Add more almond milk if mixture is too thick. Chill thoroughly.

Serve with your favorite fresh fruit.

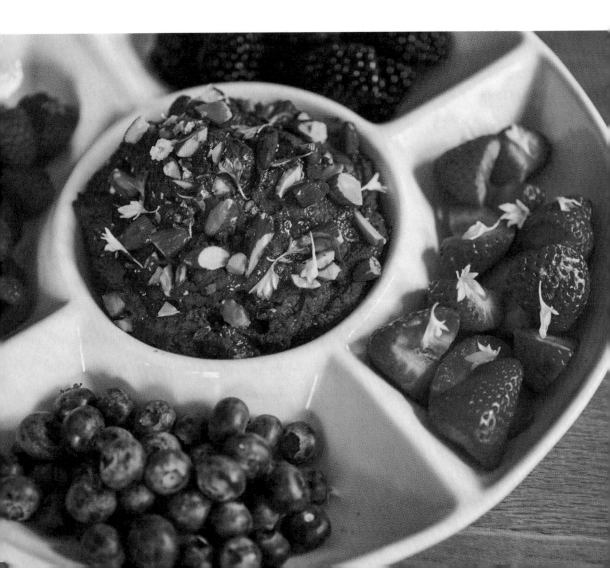

Summary Arugula and Mache Salad

Serves 2

Handful of baby arugula
Small handful of baby mache
½ lemon, freshly squeezed
1 tbsp. extra-virgin olive oil (the fancier
  the better)
Coarse sea salt to taste
Fresh cracked black pepper to taste
Pinch of roasted sesame seed
Pinch of Korean chili flake
1 c. seasonal fruit: peaches, persimmons,
  or berries, sliced or chopped
½ c. plain Greek yogurt
2 tbsp. honeycomb
¼ c. candied pecans, crushed

In a large bowl, toss arugula and mache in lemon juice and olive oil. Add pinch of salt, pepper, sesame, Korean chili flake, and sliced fruit. Spoon yogurt onto plate and place salad on top. Sprinkle the honeycomb and candied pecans on top.

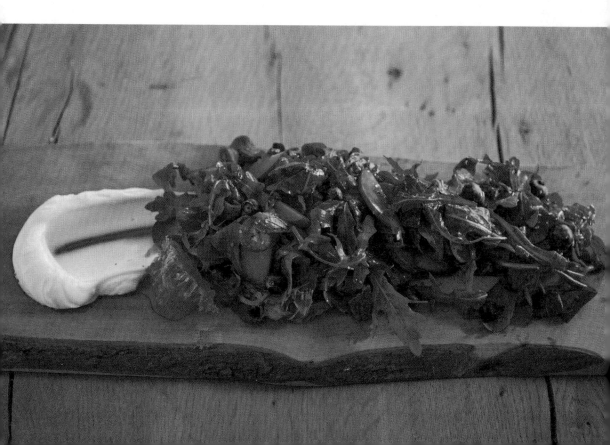

Stuffed Sweet Potato with Chorizo

Serves 4

4 medium sweet potatoes

¼ c. + 1 tbsp. extra-virgin olive oil

1 tbsp. pickling spice

1 c. plain Greek yogurt

1 clove garlic, finely minced

Kosher salt and freshly ground pepper

¼ c. golden raisins

½ lb. fresh chorizo, casings removed

2 tbsp. pine nuts

Fresh mint leaves, chopped

Preheat oven to 400°F. Bake sweet potatoes on foil-lined baking sheet 45–60 minutes, until tender. Heat 2 tbsp. olive oil in small skillet over medium-high. Add pickling spice and stir until toasted, about 1 minute. Transfer to a food processor and pulse until finely ground, about 1 minute. Transfer the spiced oil to a bowl and stir in yogurt, garlic, 1 tsp. salt, and ⅛ tsp. black pepper; set aside.

Soak raisins 10 minutes in ½ cup warm water. Meanwhile, heat 2 tbsp. olive oil in a large skillet over medium-high heat. Add chorizo and cook, stirring and breaking up meat with a wooden spoon, until browned, 5 minutes. Stir in pine nuts and cook, stirring, until lightly toasted, about 30 seconds. Transfer mixture to a bowl. Drain raisins and stir into chorizo mixture.

Split baked sweet potatoes in half. Fluff with a fork; season with salt and pepper. Top with chorizo, yogurt sauce, and mint.

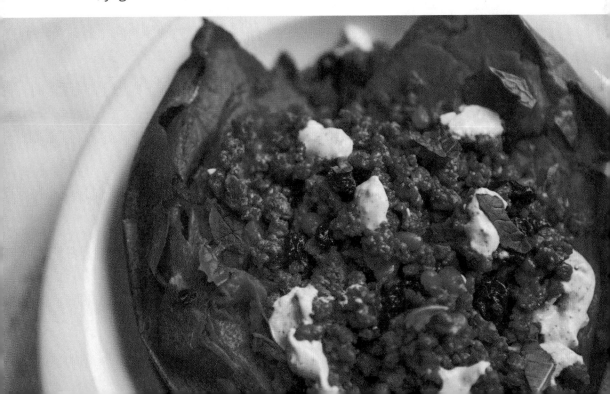

Scallion and Mint Pesto

Makes 1 cup

½ c. toasted almonds

2 garlic cloves, minced

A dozen scallions, white and light green parts only, roughly chopped

½ c. fresh basil leaves, packed

⅓ c. fresh mint leaves

⅓ c. extra-virgin olive oil

⅓ c. water

2 tsp. freshly squeezed lemon juice

1½ tsp. kosher salt

Purée everything in a blender or food processor until smooth.

Serve with cooked brown rice pasta or zucchini noodles (good for 1.5 lbs.) and with shrimp, chicken, turkey, beef, or pork.

You can also toss with 1 lb. of roasted or steamed beets for a healthy salad.

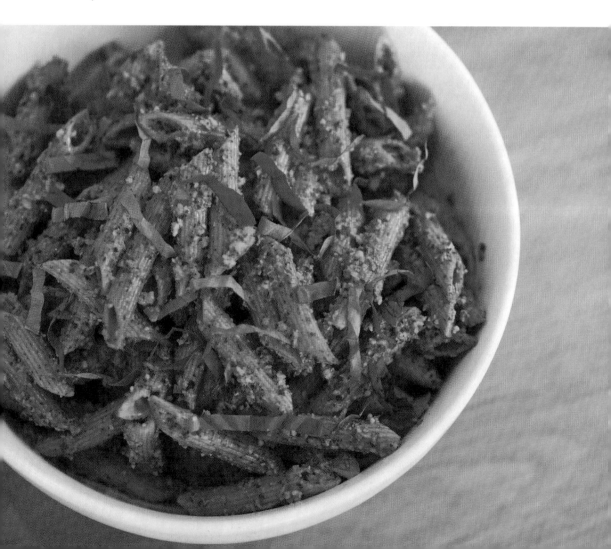

Grilled Zucchini with Blueberry Chile Salsa

Serves 6–8

1 c. blueberries

½ habanero chile (seeded for milder salsa)

¾ c. + 1 tbsp. Thai basil leaves, preferably opal basil

1 tsp. finely grated garlic

1 tsp. finely grated peeled ginger

¼ c. unseasoned rice vinegar

¼ c. purple grape juice

⅓ c. grape seed oil

3 zucchini (1.5 lb.) sliced lengthwise into ½ inch thick strips, or cut lengthwise into quartered spears

2 tbsp. extra-virgin olive oil

Kosher salt

Fresh cracked black pepper

Korean chili flakes

Roasted sesame seeds

In a food processor, combine blueberries, habanero, and ¾ c. basil, with garlic, ginger, vinegar, and grape juice. With machine on, add grape seed oil slowly until the salsa is blended but still chunky.

Light up a grill. In large bowl, toss the zucchini with the olive oil and season with salt, pepper, Korean chili flakes, and sesame seeds. Grill over moderate heat until lightly charred and tender, 1–2 minutes per side.

Transfer zucchini to a platter and garnish with the remaining 1 tbsp. of Thai basil. Drizzle salsa all over or serve on the side.

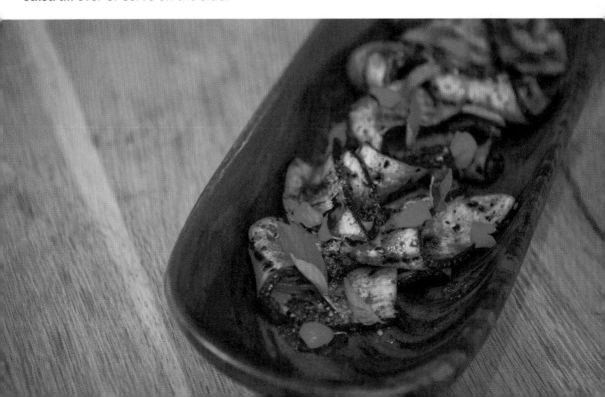

No-Bake Chocolate Peanut Butter Protein Bars
Makes 12 bars

½ c. honey

½ c. peanut butter

3 c. brown rice cereal

½ c. chopped peanuts

¼ c. protein powder

½ c. semisweet chocolate chips, chilled

Combine honey and peanut butter in saucepan; melt and stir over medium-low heat until combined. Stir in brown rice cereal, chopped peanuts, and protein powder. Add chilled chocolate chips last so they don't melt. Transfer mixture to parchment-lined 8" x 8" baking dish. Smooth a sheet of parchment paper over the top. Refrigerate 4 hours or overnight.

Mint Chocolate Smoothie
Serves 1

1 c. Greek yogurt

¼ c. fresh mint, tightly packed

1 c. almond milk

¼ c. dark chocolate chips

1 c. baby spinach

2 c. ice

Blend ingredients until smooth.

Pumpkin Smoothie Bowl

Serves 1

2 oz. fresh pumpkin or pumpkin puree

1 frozen banana, chopped

1 c. plain yogurt

½ c. almond milk

1 tsp. maple syrup

1 tsp. raw honey

Pinch of cinnamon

Pinch of ground ginger

If using fresh pumpkin, steam for 5–8 minutes; let cool 5 minutes. Blend all ingredients until smooth. Pour into a bowl and top with desired toppings. Best served chilled.

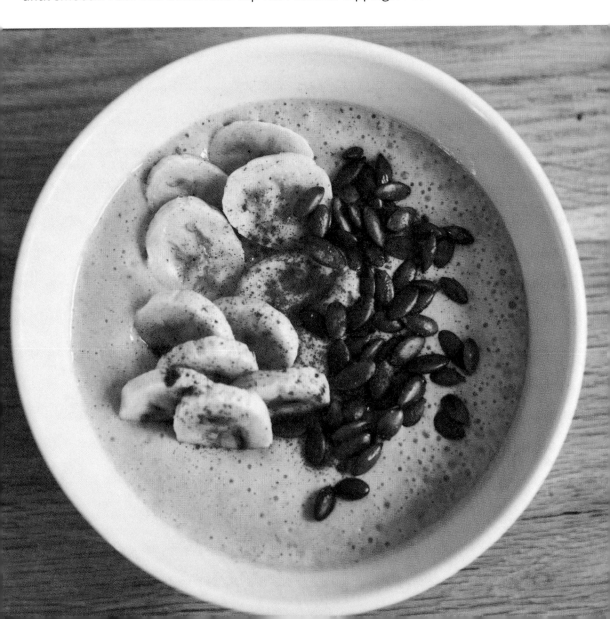

Avocado Toast with Smoked Salmon
Serves 1

1 slice country grain or sourdough bread,
  approximately ½ inch thick

Extra-virgin olive oil

½ avocado

2 slices heirloom tomato

3 slices cucumber

3 thin slices red onion

3 pieces thinly sliced smoked salmon

Freshly squeezed lemon juice to taste

Kosher salt and freshly ground black
  pepper

Lightly brush bread with olive oil and toast until golden brown. Top with avocado and mash with a fork to cover entire surface. Top with tomato, cucumber, red onion, and smoked salmon. Add lemon juice and sprinkle with salt and pepper.

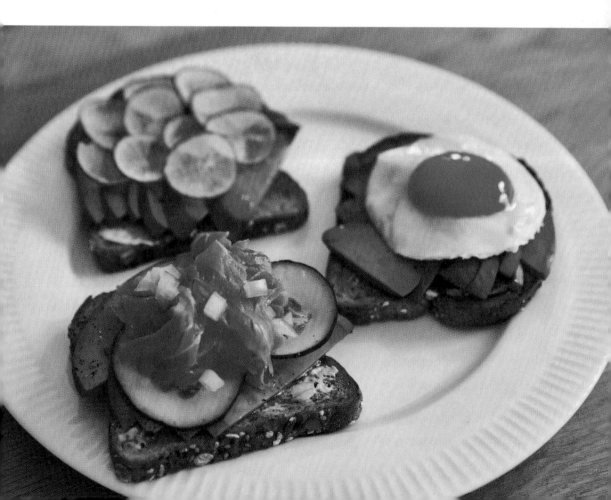

Blackberry Cashew Tarts
Makes 12

Base:
1¾ oz. walnuts
1¾ oz. almond meal
8 medjool dates, pitted
1 tbsp. coconut oil, melted

Cashew filling:
4¾ oz. unsalted cashew nuts, soaked in
  water for 1–2 hours
¼ c. milk of choice
2 tbsp. coconut oil, melted
1 tbsp, maple syrup
¼ tsp. vanilla extract

Blackberry Filling:
2⅓ oz. unsalted cashew nuts, soaked in
  water for 1–2 hours
1½ tbsp. milk of choice
3 oz. frozen blackberries, lightly thawed
2 tsp. coconut oil, melted
2 tsp. maple syrup
Finely grated zest and juice of 1 small
  orange
Extra blackberries and finely grated orange
  zest, for sprinkling (optional)

(Continued on page 288)

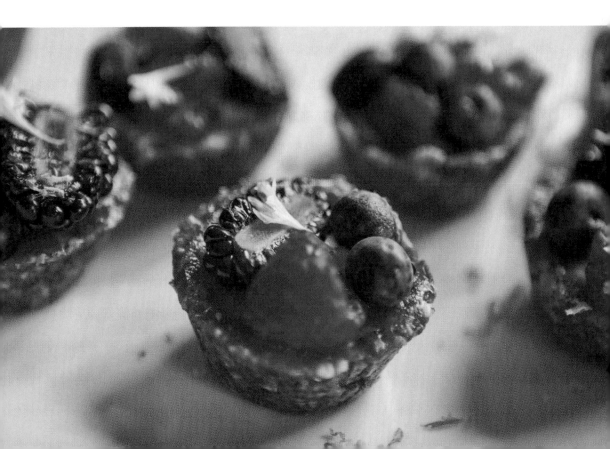

Place 12 cupcake liners in muffin tin.

Base: Place walnuts, almond meal, dates, and coconut oil in a food processor and process until crumbly. The mixture should stick together when pressed. If too dry, add up to 2 tbsp. melted coconut oil until mixture sticks together.

Press base mixture evenly into the bottom of the lined muffin cups. Refrigerate to set while you make the cashew filling.

Cashew filling: Place drained cashews, milk, coconut oil, maple syrup, and vanilla in food processor and process until smooth. Spoon evenly over base, leaving space for blackberry filling. Refrigerate while preparing blackberry filling.

Blackberry filling: Place drained cashews, milk, blackberries, coconut oil, maple syrup, and orange zest and juice in food processor and process until smooth. Spoon evenly over cashew filling.

Place muffin tin in freezer for 1–2 hours or overnight.

Remove tarts from freezer 20 minutes before serving. Top with extra blackberries and orange zest, if desired. Can be refrigerated 1–2 days or frozen up to 2 months.

THE SUPPORTER PROFILE

Familiar tastes, comfort foods, healthy but not gimmicky

Balsamic Dressing

Serves 4

½ c. balsamic vinegar
2 tbsp. brown sugar
1 tbsp. olive oil

In small saucepan, boil together vinegar and sugar to reduce by half. Cool. Then add oil and combine.

Lemon Vinaigrette

Serves 4

2 tbsp. olive oil
¼ c. apple cider vinegar
Zest of 1 lemon
1 tbsp. sugar
3 tbsp. lemon juice

Whisk together ingredients. Store in glass container.

Hawaiian Grilled Cheese

Serves 2

4 tsp. butter
4 slices white Hawaiian sweet bread
1 oz. low-fat cheddar
1 oz. provolone
2 pineapple rings

Butter bread. Place two slices on griddle over medium heat. Top each with ½ oz. cheddar, ½ oz. provolone, and 1 pineapple ring. Top with second slice of buttered bread. Cook until bread is golden and cheese is melted, about 2 to 4 minutes per side.

Grilled Chicken Bruschetta

Serves 4

¼ c. oil

Juice of 1 lemon, divided

Kosher salt

Freshly ground black pepper

1 tsp. Italian seasoning

4 boneless skinless 4 oz. chicken breasts,
  pounded to even thickness

2 oz. provolone

3 tomatoes, diced (Roma preferred)

In a small bowl, whisk together oil, half the lemon juice (about 2 tbsp.), 1 tsp. salt, ¼ tsp. pepper, and Italian seasoning. Pour over chicken in resealable plastic bag. Marinate in fridge for 30 minutes. Grill marinated chicken over medium-high heat until cooked through, 5 to 7 minutes per side. During final minutes, top each breast with ½ oz. cheese. Top chicken with diced tomatoes mixed with 2 tbsp. lemon juice, salt, and pepper.

Roasted Red Potatoes

Serves 3

1½ lb. baby red potatoes, quartered

2 tbsp. olive oil

2 tbsp. coarsely chopped fresh rosemary

Coarse salt and freshly ground pepper

Preheat oven to 450°F. In large roasting pan, toss potatoes with oil, rosemary, salt, and pepper, until evenly coated. Spread in single layer and bake 20 minutes, stirring occasionally.

Spinach Pesto Flatbread

Serves 4

½ c. pesto

2 naan flatbreads or 1 cooked thin-crust
  pizza crust

6 oz. fresh mozzarella, shredded

⅓ c. baby spinach

1 c. cherry tomatoes, halved

1 6-oz. diced, cooked chicken breast

Crushed red pepper flakes

Preheat oven to 425°F. Spread pesto evenly over flatbreads or pizza crust. Sprinkle with mozzarella, top with spinach, tomatoes, and chicken, then sprinkle with red pepper flakes. Bake on baking sheet lined with parchment paper, about 10–13 minutes, or until cheese is bubbling. Slice when slightly cooled.

Garlic Shrimp

Serves 3

3 tbsp. extra-virgin olive oil, divided

3 cloves garlic, minced

2 tsp. lime juice

½ tsp. chili powder

¼ tsp. kosher salt

⅓ c. chopped cilantro, plus more for serving

⅓ c. finely diced onion

1 lb. medium shrimp, peeled and deveined

In a small bowl, whisk together 2 tbsps. olive oil, garlic, lime juice, chili powder, salt, and cilantro. Pour over shrimp and coat thoroughly. Cover and refrigerate 10 minutes. Heat 1 tbsp. olive oil in skillet over medium-high heat. Add onions and cook until fragrant, 2 to 3 minutes. Add coated shrimp and cook on one side until pink, about 45 seconds, then flip over and cook about 1 minute more to finish. Top with extra cilantro, if desired.

Mexican Turkey and Brown Rice Skillet

Serves 4

1 lb. ground turkey

1 c. chopped onion

2 cloves garlic, minced

1 tsp. kosher salt

½ tsp. freshly ground black pepper

1 red bell pepper, diced

2 c. crushed tomatoes

2 or 3 chipotle chiles in adobo, chopped

½ c. chopped fresh cilantro, plus more for garnish

1½ c. grated low-fat cheddar

3 c. instant brown rice

Preheat oven to 375°F. Brown turkey, onion, and garlic over medium-high heat, about 5 minutes. Season with salt and pepper. Add bell pepper and cook 2 to 3 minutes more. Add tomatoes and chipotle; simmer until warmed through, 2 to 3 minutes. Stir in cilantro. Place skillet in oven, top with cheese, and bake until cheese is melted, 3 to 4 minutes. Serve on brown rice. Garnish with cilantro if desired.

Ginger Salmon

Serves 4

1 large broccoli head, cut into ½-inch-thick steaks

Extra-virgin olive oil, for drizzling

Kosher salt

Freshly ground black pepper

2 tbsp. honey

Juice of 1 lemon

1 clove garlic, grated

1¼-inch piece fresh ginger, peeled and grated

2 lb. salmon, cut into 4 pieces

2 green onions, sliced

Preheat large cast-iron grill pan. Toss broccoli with a drizzle of olive oil and season with salt and pepper. Grill broccoli until charred, about 2 minutes on each side. In a small bowl, prepare salmon glaze of honey, lemon juice, garlic, and ginger.

Rinse salmon and pat dry. Drizzle with olive oil and season with salt and pepper. Sear salmon on each side for 4 minutes. Brush on glaze and remove from grill. Serve salmon and broccoli with risotto. Garnish with green onions.

Flank Steak with Watermelon Salad

Serves 4

1 tbsp. brown sugar

1 tsp. garlic powder

1 tsp. chili powder

2 lb. flank steak

2 tbsp. balsamic vinegar

¼ c. extra-virgin olive oil

Kosher salt

Freshly ground black pepper

4 c. arugula

¼ c. chopped red onion

1 c. croutons

2 c. watermelon, cut into chunks

½ c. feta, crumbled

In a small bowl combine brown sugar, garlic powder, and chili powder. Rub mixture over steak.

Grill on high heat 5 minutes each side, then let meat rest for 3 to 4 minutes.

Prepare salad: In a large bowl combine vinegar, olive oil, salt, and pepper. Toss in arugula, onion, croutons, and watermelon. Slice the meat, and serve over salad topped with crumbled feta.

Simple Acai Smoothie Bowl

Serves 2

1 c. baby spinach

1 c. unsweetened almond milk

2 c. mixed berries

2 pkg. (3½ oz. each) unsweetened acai purée

1 large banana

Blend spinach and almond milk until smooth. Add berries, acai purée, and banana. Blend again.

Top with granola, fresh fruit, nuts, and seeds.

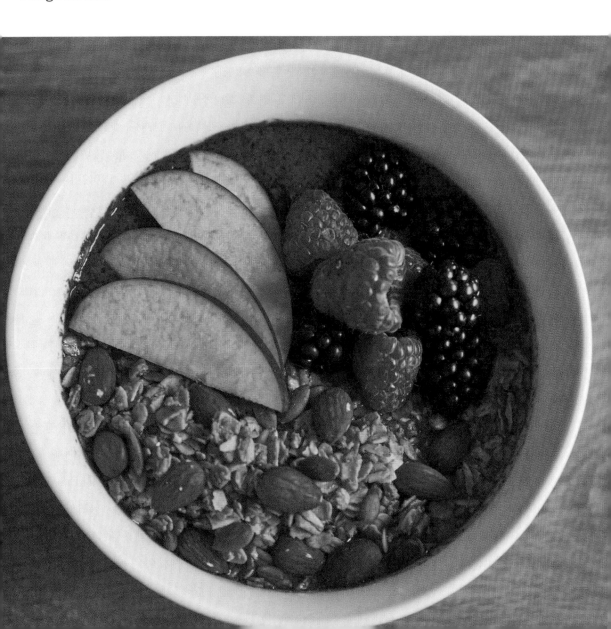

Turkey Meatballs

Serves 4

1 small onion, roughly chopped
2 garlic cloves, roughly chopped
8 fresh sage leaves
1 tbsp. fresh thyme leaves
1 tbsp. fresh rosemary leaves
¼ cup Italian parsley
1 handful of arugula, roughly chopped
1 lb. ground turkey
1 tsp. kosher salt
½ tsp. fresh cracked black pepper
4 c. Homemade Tomato Sauce

Combine onion, garlic, herbs, and arugula in food processor until very finely chopped. Transfer mixture to a large bowl, along with turkey, salt, and pepper. Use your hands to thoroughly combine all ingredients, then roll mixture into golf ball–sized meatballs.

Preheat oven to 400°F. Bake 15–20 minutes or until meatballs are firm. Toss meatballs into tomato sauce.

Homemade Tomato Sauce

2 tbsp. extra-virgin olive oil
6 garlic cloves, thinly sliced
2 28-oz. cans whole peeled tomatoes with
  juice
8 large basil leaves, torn
Salt and pepper to taste

Heat olive oil in large saucepan over low heat. Add garlic; cook for 5 minutes. Add tomatoes with their juice. Add basil leaves. Turn heat to high, bring sauce to a boil, turn heat to low, and season with salt and pepper. Simmer on low 30–45 minutes, stirring occasionally and crushing tomatoes with a wooden spoon.

Grilled Garlic-Chili Shrimp

Serves 4

1 fresh Fresno chile, seeds removed, finely minced

3 garlic cloves, finely minced

1 tbsp. coarsely ground pepper

1 tbsp. fresh lime juice

1 tsp. sesame oil

2 tbsp. vegetable oil, plus more for grill

1 lb. large shrimp, peeled, deveined

Kosher salt

Lime wedges for garnish

Fresh cilantro leaves for garnish

Crushed roasted peanuts for garnish

Korean chili flakes

Roasted sesame seeds

Whisk chile, garlic, pepper, lime juice, sesame oil, and 2 tbsps. vegetable oil in large bowl. Add shrimp and toss to coat; season with salt. Heat grill to medium-high, clean grill, and coat with oil. Grill shrimp, turning once, until cooked through and lightly charred, about 5 minutes total. Serve with lime wedges and garnish with cilantro and peanuts.

Add healthy grains and Bok Choy and Mushroom Stir-Fry (page 304) to create a bowl meal. Garnish with Korean chili flakes and sesame seeds.

Healthy Sweet Potato Wedges with Sriracha Crème Fraîche

Serves 4

3 large sweet potatoes, cut into wedges

¼ c. extra-virgin olive oil

Kosher salt

Freshly cracked pepper

Roasted sesame seeds

Korean chili flakes

½ c. crème fraîche

2 tsp. sriracha

1 tsp. fresh lemon juice

Fresh cilantro leaves for garnish

Preheat oven to 400°F. Place sweet potatoes on baking sheet and drizzle with oil; season with salt, pepper, sesame, and Korean chili flakes. Toss to coat and spread out in a single layer. Roast until golden brown and slightly crispy, 25–35 minutes.

Mix crème fraîche, sriracha, and lemon juice in a small bowl. Serve with potatoes, and garnish with cilantro.

Melon and Cucumber Salad
Serves 4

½ c. extra-virgin olive oil

¼ c. champagne vinegar

1 tsp. ground coriander

1 tsp. kosher salt

¼ tsp. freshly cracked black pepper

⅛ tsp. ground cardamom

½ cantaloupe, cut into 1-inch pieces

1 cucumber, sliced ½ inch thick

2 Fresno chilies, thinly sliced

½ c. roasted pepitas (pumpkin seeds)

¼ c. fresh cilantro, chopped

¼ c. fresh mint leaves, chopped

Sumac (tarty and citrusy spice from Middle East)

Whisk oil, vinegar, coriander, salt, pepper, and cardamom in large bowl. Add cantaloupe, cucumber, and chiles; toss to coat. Let sit uncovered 15 minutes. Add pumpkin seeds, cilantro, and mint to salad and toss gently to combine. Garnish with sumac.

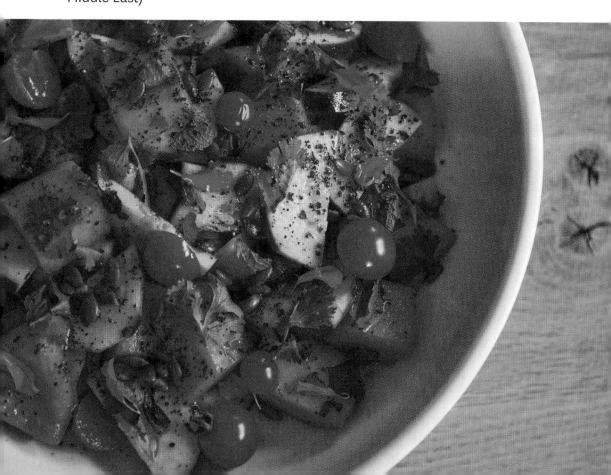

Chocolate Protein Pancakes

Serves 2

1 large banana

2 whole eggs or egg whites

2 tbsp. almond milk

⅓ c. almond flour

3 tbps. chocolate protein powder or fresh cacao powder

⅛ tsp. baking powder

¼ tsp. ground cinnamon

Add all the ingredients (wet first, then dry) to a food processor or blender. Blend until smooth and the consistency of pancake batter. Heat a large skillet to medium heat.

Spray with cooking spray. Add batter to the pan. Cook each side of the pancake 1–2 minutes. Serve with fresh fruit and 3 tbsp. maple syrup.

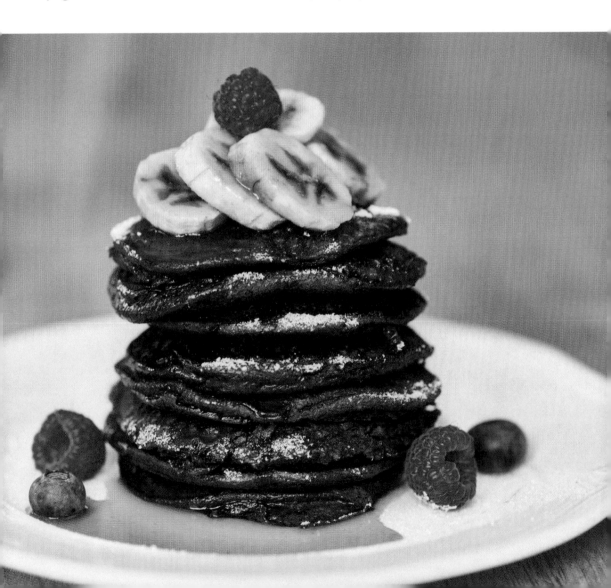

Simple Beet Salad

Serves 1

¼ c. roasted beets

3 c. arugula

¼ c. cooked quinoa

Extra-virgin olive oil to taste

Lemon juice to taste

¼ avocado

1 oz. goat cheese

1 tbsp. toasted pepitas

Honeycomb

Toss beets with arugula, quinoa, olive oil, and lemon juice. Top with avocado, goat cheese, and pepitas and serve with honeycomb.

Zucchini/Blueberry Muffins

Makes 12 (Freeze them for a quick brekkie or snack!)

1 ½ c. whole-wheat flour or almond flour

1 tsp. baking soda

1 tsp. cinnamon

¼ tsp. salt

1 c. shredded zucchini (about 1 medium zucchini)

½ c. maple syrup (or honey)

1 tsp. vanilla extract

¼ tsp. almond extract

2 tbsp. olive oil

⅓ c. unsweetened applesauce

1 egg

¼ c. unsweetened almond milk (or any milk)

¾ c. fresh or frozen blueberries

Preheat oven to 350°F. Prepare a 12-cup muffin pan with nonstick cooking spray or muffin liners. Combine dry ingredients in a large bowl. Combine wet ingredients (including zucchini) in separate medium bowl; add to dry ingredients and stir until just combined. Gently fold in blueberries. Fill muffin tins ¾ full and bake 19–22 minutes, or until toothpick inserted comes out clean.

Red Beet Smoothie
Serves 2

1 small apple, cored.
1 raw red beet, washed, peeled. Do not use cooked.
1 handful blueberries or raspberries
1 handful kale
¼ c. pineapple
½ navel orange peeled
½ c. ice
½ c. ice water
1 tbsp. flaxseed (optional)

Layer every ingredient into a food processor or blender. Adjust amount of water so that ingredients mix smoothly.

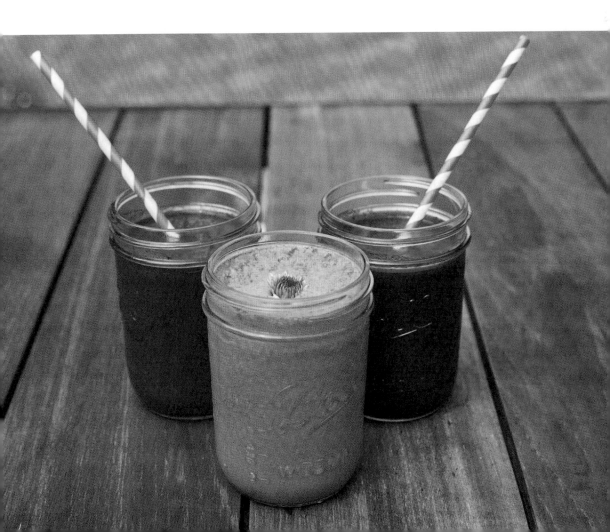

Stuffed Avocado with Corn Salsa

Serves 2

1 avocado, halved
1½ c. corn
⅓ c. red onion, diced
¼ c. cilantro, minced
½ tsp. cumin
½ tsp. salt
1 jalapeño, minced
2 tbsp. lime juice
1 red tomato, cored, diced

After halving avocado, scoop out some of the pitted area to widen the "bowl." Mix all ingredients in a bowl and scoop into avocado halves.

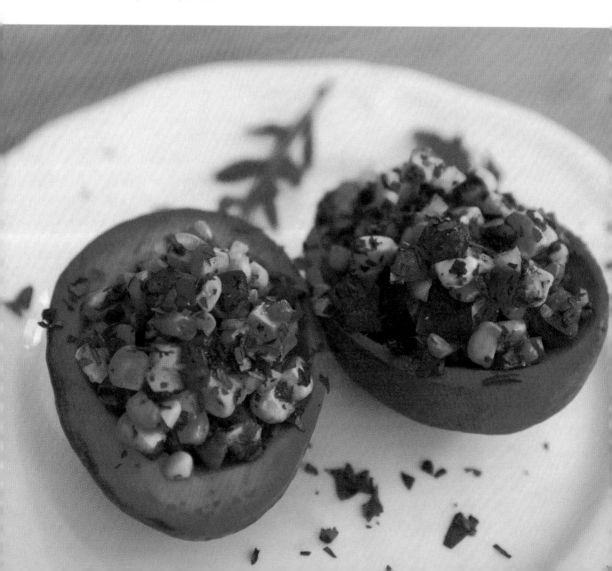

Stuffed Avocado with Salmon

1 avocado, halved
6 oz. salmon, baked
¼ c. red bell pepper, diced
1 tbsp. jalapeño, minced

¼ c. cilantro leaves, roughly chopped
1 tbsp. lime juice
Kosher salt and pepper to taste
1 tbsp. low-fat mayo (optional)

After halving avocado, scoop out some of the pitted area to widen the "bowl." With a fork, mash the scooped avocado in a medium-size mixing bowl Add the salmon, bell pepper, jalapeño, and cilantro to bowl. Pour lime juice over. Stir until well mixed.

Scoop into the avocado bowls; season with salt and pepper.

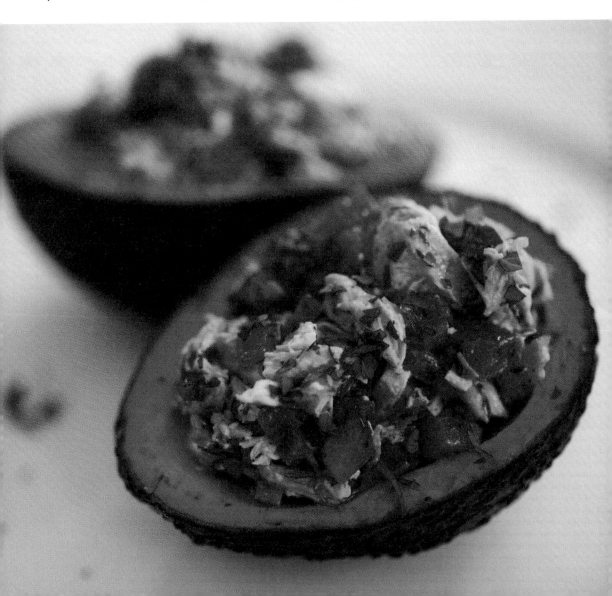

Raspberry Chia Bowl

Serves 4

2 c. unsweetened almond milk

2 tsp. raw honey

½ c. chia seeds

2 c. fresh raspberries (reserve 8 for garnish)

Fresh mint leaves for garnish

Combine almond milk, honey, chia seeds, and raspberries in medium bowl; mix well.

Cover and refrigerate 4 hours or overnight, mixing after 2 hours. Place chia seed mixture in small serving glasses or bowls; garnish with raspberries and mint leaves.

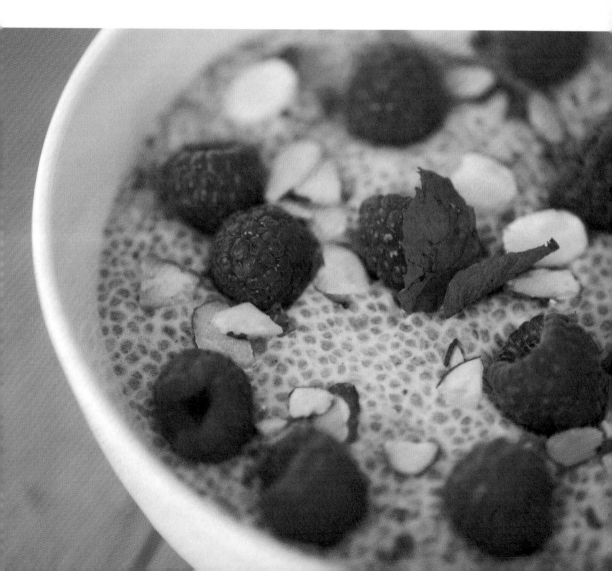

Stuffed Pita with Greek Salad
Serves 4-6

Pita bread
1 lb. baby green mix
2 large heirloom tomatoes, sliced
1 small red onion, sliced
1 cucumber, sliced
Dash of smoked sea salt

Tzatziki Sauce

1 cucumber, grated
2 garlic cloves, grated
2 c. plain Greek yogurt
2 tbsp. finely chopped dill
2 tbsp. fresh lemon juice
2 tbsp. olive oil
Kosher salt and black pepper

Preheat oven to 400°F. Cut pitas in half, place on cookie sheet, and bake 5-6 minutes. Turn bread over and bake for 3-5 minutes longer until golden brown. Stuff pitas with toppings evenly. Serve with tzatziki sauce.

Mix cucumber, garlic, yogurt, dill, lemon juice, and oil in a medium bowl; season with salt and pepper. Cover and let sit at room temperature for one hour, until flavors meld. Tzatziki can be made 1 day ahead. Chill.

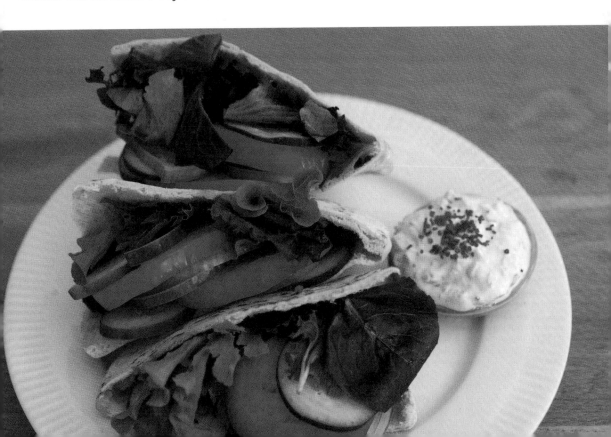

Bok Choy and Mushroom Stir-Fry
Serves 4

1 lb. bok choy, rinsed and drained
1½ tbsp. extra-virgin olive oil
3 cloves garlic, minced
4 oz. mushrooms, cremini or portobello, sliced
Salt and pepper to taste

Rinse bok choy with cold water. Cut and remove lower part of stems. Cut the bigger leaves lengthwise to halves, set aside.

Heat oil in large skillet on medium-high, add garlic, and stir-fry until aromatic. Add mushrooms and stir for about 2 minutes, then add bok choy. Add a pinch of salt and continue to stir-fry until the leaves are wilted but stems remain crisp. Turn off heat and serve immediately.

Salad Pizza
Serves 4

1 pack premade pizza dough (whole-wheat or gluten-free)
1 lb. baby greens
1 pint cherry tomatoes, halved
Shaved Parmesan
Balsamic vinaigrette

Balsamic Vinaigrette
Makes about 1 cup
¼ tsp. red chili flakes
1 garlic clove, finely grated
¼ c. balsamic vinegar
¼ c. Greek yogurt (optional)
3 tbsp. olive oil
1 tsp. honey
1 tsp. kosher salt

Preheat oven 400°F. Bake pizza dough 15–20 minutes. Toss greens, tomatoes, and 4 tbsp. dressing. Top baked dough; garnish with shaved Parmesan.

Mix chili flakes, garlic, vinegar, oil, honey, and salt in a pint jar, seal and shake vigorously until dressing is smooth and no lumps of yogurt remain, about 20 seconds. Dressing can be made 3 days ahead. Cover and chill.

THE PLANNER PROFILE

Nutritious, balanced, healthy, and palate-pleasing

Avocado and Beet Hummus Toast

Serves 1

1 slice bread
2 tbsp. beet hummus (below)
⅛ avocado, sliced
Microgreens
1 tbsp. goat cheese
1 chicken-apple sausage
1 c. blackberries

Beet Hummus:
Serves 4
1 medium beet, cooked
10 oz. plain hummus

Layer toasted bread with beet hummus, avocado, microgreens, and goat cheese. Serve with breakfast sausage and blackberries.

For the Beet Hummus: Puree everything in blender.

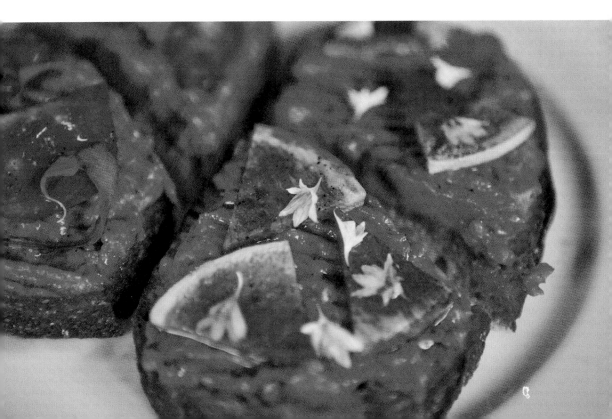

Cheese Tortellini with Ground Beef

Serves 1

3 oz. lean ground beef
1 garlic clove, minced
⅛ tsp. red pepper flakes
1 tsp. olive oil
½ c. cooked tortellini
1 c. baby spinach
sea salt
pepper
parsley

Brown ground beef, season to liking, and set aside. In a medium pan over low heat, sauté garlic and red pepper flakes in olive oil. Add cooked pasta and ground beef. Toss in spinach gently; season with salt and pepper. Garnish with chopped parsley.

Cinnamon French Toast

Serves 1

1 whole egg + 2 egg whites
1 tbsp. milk
⅛ tsp. cinnamon
⅛ tsp. maple syrup
⅛ tsp. vanilla
2 slices cinnamon swirl bread
2 tbsp. light whipped cream

Whisk egg, egg whites, milk, cinnamon, maple syrup, and vanilla in small bowl. Coat bread slices in batter. Cook on skillet over medium heat until golden brown. Top with whipped cream.

Beef and Broccoli

Serves 2

4 oz. sirloin, sliced
½ c. chopped sweet onion
1 tbsp. minced garlic
½ c. beef broth
2 c. fresh or frozen broccoli florets
2 tsp. cornstarch
½ tbsp. brown sugar
½ tsp. garlic powder

Coat skillet with cooking spray and heat over medium. Add beef, onion, and minced garlic; stir-fry until brown. Remove the beef to a plate and keep warm. Add half the broth and broccoli to pan. Cover and simmer until broccoli is tender-crisp. Stir cornstarch, brown sugar, and garlic powder into remaining broth until smooth; add to pan. Cook until mixture begins to thicken, stirring constantly. Return beef to mixture, stir, and serve over rice.

Sautéed Shrimp

Serves 4

1 tbsp. olive oil
1 small onion, chopped
1 28 oz. can diced tomatoes, drained
¾ c. pitted green olives
½ c. dry white wine
½ tsp. sea salt
¼ tsp. pepper
1 lb. shrimp, peeled and deveined

Heat oil over medium-high heat. Add onion and cook about 4 minutes. Add tomatoes, olives, wine, salt, and pepper. Simmer, stirring occasionally until slightly thickened, about 4–6 minutes. Add shrimp and cover. Cook 3–5 minutes or until shrimp turns opaque. Serve with couscous.

Orange Cantaloupe Smoothie

Serves 1

1 c. low-fat vanilla yogurt
½ c. fresh orange juice
½ c. sliced cantaloupe
4 ice cubes, crushed, or as needed

Blend ingredients until smooth.

Kalifornia Smoothie

Serves 2

2 c. kale, stems removed
1 c. water
2 oranges, peeled
½ cup pineapple
1 c. chopped mango
2 tbsp. chia seeds

Blend kale, water, and oranges until smooth. Add pineapple, mango, and chia seeds and blend again.

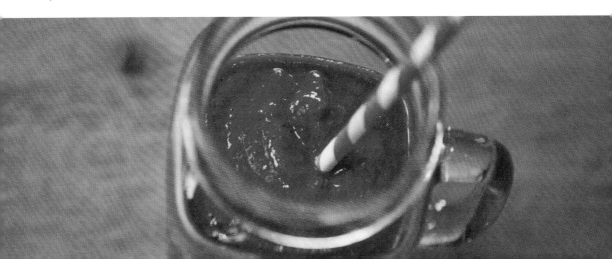

Miso Crunch Bowl
Serves 2

1 c. cooked healthy grains (quinoa, farro, barley, wild rice, or brown rice)

1 c. swiss chard or spinach, thinly sliced

1 c. green cabbage, thinly sliced

¼ c. carrots, julienned

¼ c. edamame

4 tbsp. miso-lime dressing (below)

½ lb. cooked shrimp, marinated with salt, pepper, sesame, Korean chili flake, and sesame oil

1 avocado, cut in half

2 tbsp. fresh cilantro leaves

2 tbsp. scallions, thinly sliced

1 tbsp. toasted black sesame

Divide grains into two bowls. Toss swiss chard, cabbage, carrots, and edamame in a bowl with the dressing. Place atop grains. Add shrimp and avocado and garnish with cilantro, scallions, and black sesame.

Creamy Miso Dressing
Makes 1 cup

4½ tbsp. light yellow miso

4½ tbsp. raw honey

3 tbsp. rice vinegar or wine vinegar

3 tbsp. yellow mustard

Whisk ingredients in a bowl until they are well combined and the miso has dissolved.

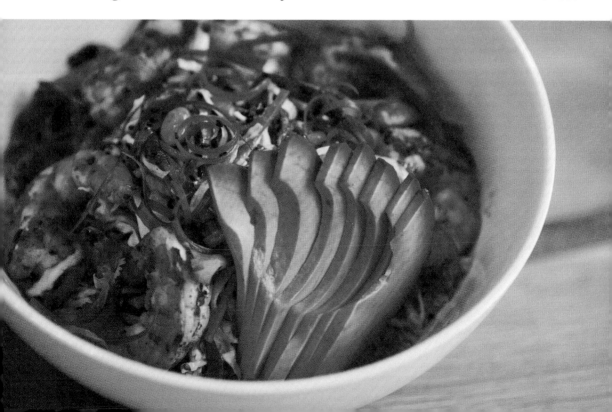

Quinoa

Serves 2

1 c. quinoa
1 ¾ c. water
Natural kosher salt

Rinse quinoa. Place in a pot with water and a big pinch of salt over high heat. Bring quinoa to a boil, lower heat, cover, and cook gently until liquid is absorbed, 12–15 minutes. Turn off heat; let quinoa sit for at least 5 minutes before fluffing with a fork.

Posole with Hominy

Serves 4

6 tomatillos, outer skin and stems removed, roughly chopped
1 large red onion, peeled and roughly chopped
2 jalapeños, roughly chopped (seeded for milder taste)
Kosher salt
Extra-virgin olive oil
4 c. vegetable stock
3 large sprigs of cilantro
1 28-oz. can hominy, drained and rinsed

For garnish:

1 ripe avocado, diced
⅓ c. fresh cilantro leaves
2 scallions, thinly sliced
2 radishes, thinly sliced
1 lime, cut into wedges

Preheat oven to 450°F. On a sheet pan, toss the tomatillos, onions, and jalapeños with a large pinch of salt and enough olive oil to coat. Roast, stirring now and then, until soft and slightly browned, about 20 minutes.

Transfer roasted vegetables to a powerful blender. Add 1 cup of stock and puree until smooth (be very careful when blending hot ingredients). Transfer mixture to a large pot along with the rest of the stock, cilantro, and the hominy. Bring to a boil, lower heat, and simmer 15 minutes, or until all flavors come together. Season to taste with salt.

Remove cilantro and garnish as you like with avocado, cilantro leaves, scallions, radishes, and/or lime wedges.

Coconut Creamed Spinach

Serves 2

1 tbsp. extra-virgin olive oil
1 garlic clove, finely minced
½ shallot, finely minced
5 oz. baby spinach leaves
4 tbsp. light coconut milk
½ tsp. mild curry powder
Salt to taste
Freshly cracked black pepper

Heat olive oil over medium in large sauté pan. Add garlic and shallot. Cook until fragrant, about 1 minute. Add spinach and stir around until it begins to wilt. Add coconut milk, curry powder, salt, and pepper. Stir until combined, about 1 minute.

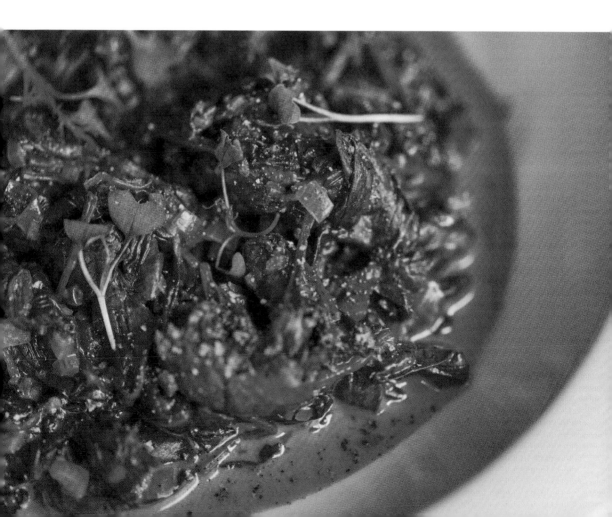

Mushroom Frittata
Serves 6

3 tbsp. extra-virgin olive oil

2 shallots, finely minced

2 garlic cloves, finely minced

1 tbsp. fresh thyme, finely minced

3 c. mixed coarsely chopped mushrooms, such as chanterelle, portobello, crimini, and maitakes

6 large eggs

2 tbsp. fresh parsley, finely chopped

¼ tsp. kosher salt

⅛ tsp. freshly cracked pepper

1 tbsp. fresh chives, finely chopped

Heat 2 tbsp. oil in nonstick skillet over medium-low heat. Add shallots, garlic, and thyme. Sauté gently for about 5 minutes, until translucent but not browned. Add mushrooms and sauté 4–5 minutes, until just starting to release their juices. Remove from heat. Crack the eggs into a large bowl with parsley, salt, and pepper. Add mushroom mixture to eggs and stir. Wipe skillet clean. Heat remaining tbsp. oil in skillet and pour in mixture. Cook over medium heat for 8–10 minutes until bottom is set. Transfer skillet to a preheated broiler and cook 2–3 minutes until top is set and spotted brown. Let cool and serve room temperature. Garnish with fresh chives.

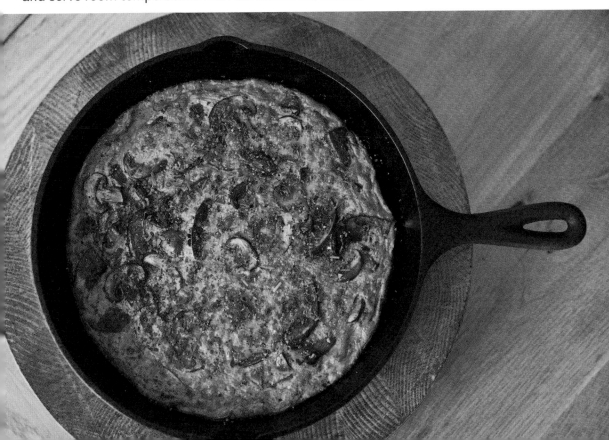

Parfait

Serves 1

½ c. Greek coconut yogurt

¼ c. crumbled angel food cake

¼ c. raspberries, blueberries,
  blackberries, bananas, strawberries

1 tbsp. coconut whipped cream

Coconut Whipped Cream

Makes 1 cup

1 c. coconut cream full-fat (refrigerate can
  overnight)

3–4 tbsp. coconut sugar

½ tsp. vanilla extract

Put ¼ cup yogurt into small mason jar. Top with crumbled angel food cake, then ¼ c. yogurt, top with fresh fruit, and garnish with coconut whipped cream.

For the Coconut Whipped Cream: Place mixing bowl in freezer 2 hours before whipping. Open refrigerated can, discard liquid, and place coconut solids in chilled bowl. Whip until fluffy. Add coconut sugar and vanilla; whip until smooth. Refrigerate until chill and firm. Serve at room temperature.

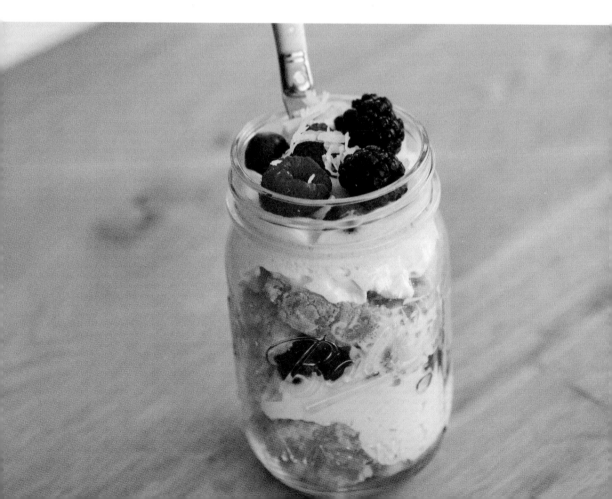

Zucchini Hummus

Serves 8

2 medium zucchini, peeled and chopped
½ c. tahini
⅓ c. fresh lemon juice
⅓ c. olive oil
3 garlic cloves
1 ½ tsp. cumin
Kosher salt and black pepper to taste

Combine all ingredients in a food processor until smooth.

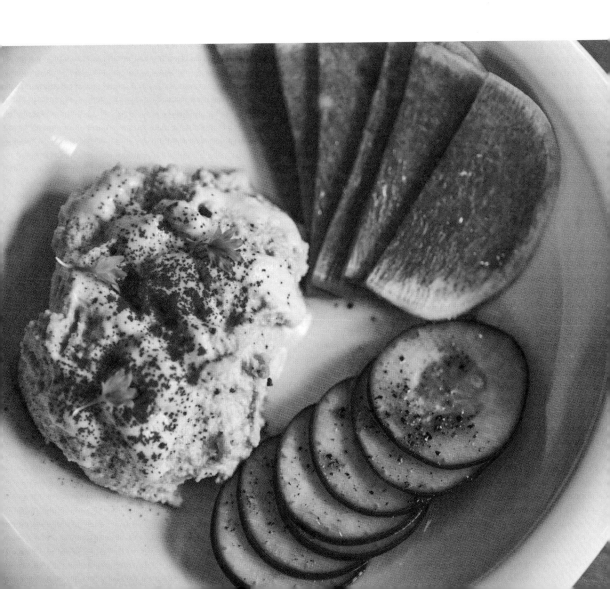

Snacks for everybody!

Because I'm a binge-monster if I get too hungry, I'm a big believer in healthy snacks. The following are great options for small meals or in-between healthy meals.

Sweet and Salty

Fruit & Nuts
1 serving any fruit
¼ c. mixed nuts

Pear & Cheese
Pear
1 String Cheese

Apple & Cheese
Green Apple
½ oz. Parmesan, sliced paper thin

For Breakfast Lovers

Egg & Mini Roll
1 hard-boiled egg
1 mini whole-wheat roll
Mustard

Yogurt & Bran Cereal
½ c. All-Bran cereal
5 oz. Greek yogurt
½ c. berries

Overnight Oats
Combine and let sit overnight:
½ c. steel-cut oats
½ c. milk
½ tsp. vanilla extract
½ tsp. cinnamon
2 tsp. honey

Top with:
½ c. berries
Chopped nuts

Sweet Snacks

Yogurt and Berries
5 oz. vanilla Greek yogurt
½ c. blueberries

Cottage Cheese and Berries
4 oz. cottage cheese
½ c. berries

Apple & Nut Butter
Apple
2 tbsp. almond butter

Protein Smoothie
6 oz. rice milk
2 scoops vanilla protein powder
½ c. frozen fruit

Banana & Peanut Butter
Banana
2 tbsp. peanut butter

More like a Mini Meal

Feta Pita Salad

1 whole-wheat mini pita

1 oz. feta

Lettuce and tomatoes

Chicken Wrap

1 oz. shredded chicken

1 oz. shredded cheese

Lettuce for wrap

Baked Yams

4–5 oz. yam

1 oz. protein

Veggie & Bean Soup

1 cup (Healthy Choice Country Vegetable)

Mini Quesadilla

1 corn tortilla

1 oz. Mexican cheese

Salsa

Caprese Salad

2 oz. fresh mozzarella

Cherry tomatoes

Fresh basil

2 oz. red wine vinegar

Crackers & Egg Salad

2 Wasa crackers

½ c. Trader Joe's Spicy Ranchero Egg White Salad

Falafel Pita

1 mini wheat pita

1–2 falafel

Cherry tomatoes

Lettuce

2 tbsp. tzatziki

Just One Ingredient

Edamame

1 cup in pods

Jerky

2 oz. any type

Three Bean Salad

½ c. Trader Joe's prepared
(technically three ingredients, but . . .)

Popcorn

1 Snack Pack

V8 Vegetable Juice

5½ oz., low sodium

Celery, pepper, and hot sauce optional

Dippables

Peppers & Tzatziki
Sliced red peppers
¼ c. tzatziki

Veggies & Yogurt Dip
Jicama, pepper strips, cucumber sticks
2 tbsp. Greek yogurt dip

Veggies & Tzatziki
Vegetable Sticks
¼ c. tzatziki

Carrots & Hummus
Handful baby carrots
4 tbsp. hummus

Packable Snacks

Lara Bar
PureFit Bar
KIND Bar plus Protein
Single Serving pack trail mix (¼ c.)

CHRISTINE'S FAVE GO-TO, GO-ANYWHERE SNACKS

Watermelon jerky

Meat and veggie bar (yes, that's literally it—delish!)

Grab-and-go hummus

Quinoa cups flavored with artichoke & roasted peppers, or mango & jalapeño (yummy!)

Flavored oils: Olive, walnut, sesame

> ***Pro tip:*** Get a mini spray can, keep in your car and add it to pita, veggies, or anything else!

Quinoa chocolate snacks

Botanical chocolate: cacao bars made with turmeric, ginger, and cinnamon (more nutrients, tastes great!)

Garlic-pepper cashews

RX bars (great protein source, and made with five or fewer ingredients!)

Sunflower cinnamon bites

On-the-go crunchy nut butters

Savory coconut chips

Superfood kale popcorn

Peanut butter in powder form (mix with water)

Watermelon water

Apples, bananas, oranges!

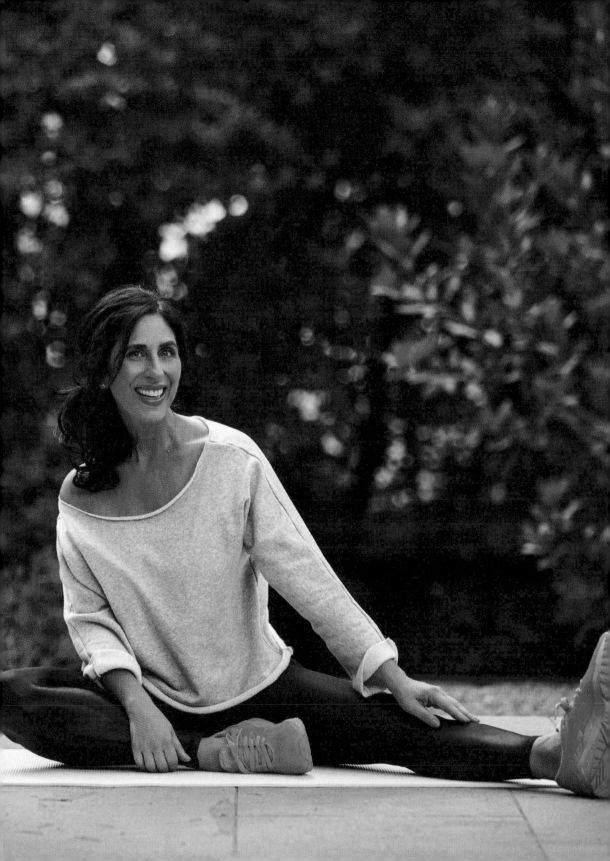

Glory Days!

■■■

Somewhere in this book, I had to lay some '80s on you.

YES, I KNOW: Everyone thinks "their" teen decade was best, but come on! The '80s! Off-the-shoulders tees, leg warmers, bodysuits cut up to *there,* big cars (screw the energy crisis), *Sixteen Candles, Breakfast Club, Dirty Dancing,* and oh my God, *What a feeling!*

For 30 years I've been completely in love with all of it, despite the fact that *during* the '80s I was completely and utterly insane.

You know that story by now. The Apple-Jacks diet, the triple StairMaster sessions, the unrelenting sense that I was irredeemably flawed and doomed to unhappiness because I had a belly and a few pounds I didn't want.

So glad *that's* over. But here's the thing. I have no regrets. That crazy teenage Christine is the whole reason I've been on this wonderful journey. If she hadn't been passionate, persistent, unrelenting and willing to try *everything,* I would have been stuck in a permanent state of *meh.* I would not have cared about myself enough to seek out the real source of happiness—which is living my best life, every day and with every action I take.

So, yes, the '80s is the soundtrack of my life. In my mind, I'm an improbably gorgeous steel worker writhing on stage under a key-lit shower of water. Or I'm a skinny blonde in a black spandex catsuit flirting with John Travolta. *Tell me about it, stud.* (The '80s Travolta, thank you.)

But in my heart I'm centered and grounded, and living with the self-acceptance I never dreamed I'd have. And yes, I still build castles in the air, but now I put foundations under them.

So I'm going to leave you with three of my favorite motivational techniques that have helped keep me moving forward, every day, every year. I hope they'll inspire you, too.

1) My personal Best Life List.

It's what I require daily to live at my strongest, healthiest, and most successful.

1) **Keep a strong body and a light heart.** When I work out, I lock my problems and worries into my mental file cabinet. No negative thoughts allowed! *And I always find a way to bring the FUN!*

2) **Keep the goal flexible.** Some days I want to go for a personal goal: *I'm going to run an eight-minute mile for five miles.* (Yes, that's fast. I *am* fast!) But some days I just want to move. No goal, no measurement.

3) **Stay ethical.** I do my best to honor others and keep my word. And I don't cheat myself, either. I don't say I ran three miles when I really ran two and a half. Keeping myself honest keeps me from rationalizing, excuse making, and defending—all of which rob me of my precious energy.

4) **Stay in acceptance.** The credits never roll when it comes to living a healthy life. I'll be doing this into my eighties, people! Moving with purpose and eating well are as necessary as sun and rain. So why not just keep finding ways to make it easier for myself, and my clients?

5) **Look as good as I can.** Letting myself go never makes me feel good. I like to feel I'm presenting my best self.

6) **Maintain discipline.** And by that I do not mean strapping on the leather and brandishing a whip on myself (although that *would* be very '80s). I mean stating my desires and taking small steps toward them daily. Even if it's just five minutes a day, any time spent working toward a goal ensures that I *can* get it done.

Now it's your turn. I invite you to create your own Best Life List here. Print it, laminate it, stick it in your purse or pocket, and use it as your own motivational go-to.

2) My favorite motivational sayings.

On those tougher days, I find these words ear-worming into my conscious.

"The secret to change is to focus all your energy not on fighting the old but on creating the new."

—*Socrates*

"The question isn't who's going to let me. It's who's going to stop me."

—*Ayn Rand, novelist, founder of Objectivism*

"When your legs get tired, run with your heart."

—*Boston Marathon slogan*

"If you're trying, you're never failing."

—*Anonymous*

"Done is better than perfect."

—*Gary Mack, sports psychologist*

"It's not how you started, it's how you finish."

—*Joel Osteen, motivational speaker and author*

"I will not let one bad meal or one bad day get in the way of accomplishing my goals."

—*Christine Lusita*

3) My theme song!

Hasn't stopped motivating me yet! This song is '80s to its ripped-shoulder core. It's about choosing your best life, and to me, choice is freedom. And freedom is . . . well, it's break-dancing and roller-skating and Dolphin shorts and Flashdance. It's big like Morgan Fairchild's hair and loud like a Guns N' Roses concert. It's hungry like the wolf. It's a feeling, people! And on that note, I invite you to dance with me to your best life . . .

Take your passion and make it happen, baby!

XOXO always,
Coach Christine

What a feelin'

First when there's nothing
But a slow glowing dream
That your fear seems to hide
Deep inside your mind

All alone I have cried
Silent tears full of pride
In a world made of steel
Made of stone

Well, I hear the music
Close my eyes, feel the rhythm
Wrap around
Take a hold of my heart

What a feeling
Bein's believin'
I can have it all
Now I'm dancing for my life

Take your passion
And make it happen
Pictures come alive
You can dance right through your life

Now I hear the music
Close my eyes, I am rhythm
In a flash
It takes hold of my heart

What a feeling
Bein's believin'
I can have it all
Now I'm dancing for my life

Take your passion
And make it happen
Pictures come alive
You can dance right through your life

What a feeling!!

ARTIST: IRENE CARA / 1983

Acknowledgments

My heart feels so many things as I write this: awe, inspiration, and endless, endless gratitude. This book had been my dream for many years, and so many wonderful people helped me make it come true.

First, my thanks to my editor, Diane Cyr, who so beautifully caught every one of my words, thoughts, and ideas, no matter how fast or wide I threw them out. Your fun, wit, dedication, heart, and talent have inspired me beyond words. You are my extraordinaire!

To the gifted Adam Fogelson, longtime client and mentor, who gave me the support and guidance to turn my what-ifs into rock-solid reality. Your immense talent inspires me! My gratitude to you and Hillary is immeasurable.

To Helen Adams Zimmermann, beloved agent. Your dedication knows no bounds. I adore you and thank you!

To my team at Skyhorse Publishing, especially Leah Zarra and Abigail Gehring: thank you for making the book a reality! xo

To David Avrin, marketing genius, who listened to my ideas and showed me how to make them sing. Thank you for being my human Waze—the one who always knows where to go and the best way to get there!

To Niece Pecenka, my beautiful workout guru, and Kirstin Hill, super-smart RDN. Thank you both so much for being a joy to work with!

To Matt Beard, my amazing photographer, whose creativity and talent have made this book look almost as yummy as the food itself. I'm still in awe. You are a superstar!

To Chef Micko Ortiz: I'm so lucky to collaborate with someone who knows how to make healthy eating so simple and delicious—you rock!

To my wonderful community at the UCLA Mindful Awareness Research Center, particularly Mitra Manesh, Kelly Barron, and my loving teacher, Diana Winston. You have given me so much hope and wisdom throughout my yo-yo journey, and always inspired me to become the best version of myself. I cannot thank you enough for your peace, support, and love.

To my BFF Louise Hill. You give me such confidence! Thank you for listening, for loving, and for being with me every step of the way. I love you to pieces.

To Marta Martin, my fun-loving friend, and terrific '80s dance partner!

To dear Flavio Marenco and Jessica Oifer, my loving guides, who have helped me see that I truly am a diamond in the rough who just needed a little polishing.

To Brooke Goldstein, my social media maven, who has helped pull it all together at the start of this project. And to Ed Borquist, my fabulous graphic designer. And to Murray Smith for her elegant visual edits. Mmmwah!

To Michele Mastriacni at bookchick.net, Margaret Doughtery, and Kate Zendall: a big thanks for your wonderful contributions!

To my mom, Carol, my dad, Rich, and my sister, Kim—and to my loving in-laws, Carmela and Tom: thank you for always believing in me and making me think I can do anything. I love you all deeply!

To Lily, the four-legged love of my life. Your smiles and kisses make my world.

To God, who makes everything possible.

And always to Jay, my uber-supportive, fun-loving, adorable husband, and the backbone of my life. Thank you for always saying, "You got this." The last twenty-plus years have been the best of my life, and I love you so very much.

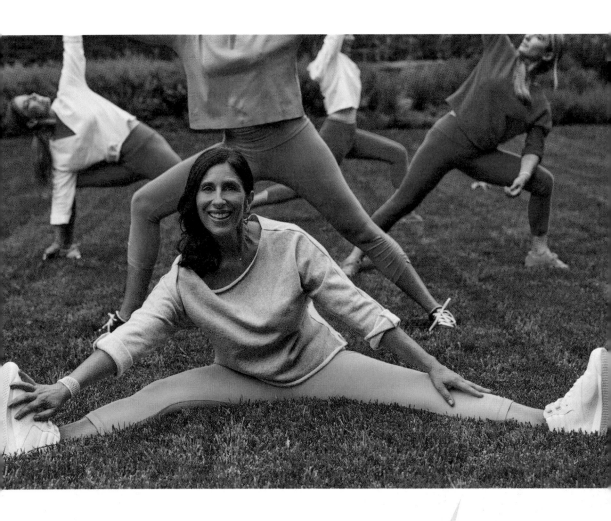

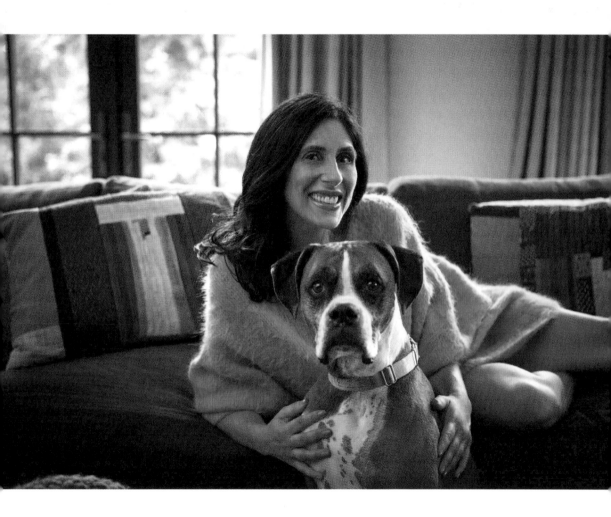

About the Author

Diet and fitness expert Christine Lusita CPT, CHC, is a celebrated health coach, mindfulness educator, behavior change specialist, nutritionist, and a Polestar Pilates instructor.

For the past fifteen years, Christine has shared her "do what feels good" philosophy in private practice with Fortune 100 CEOs, moms, families, athletes, and everyone in between. In addition to collaborating with several major brands such as Planet Fitness, POM, and Reebok, Christine also been featured on such national media outlets as *The Today Show*, *Steve Harvey*, EXTRA TV, KTLA, and ABC.

Christine's passion has been to help people discover their true *Right Fit* for leading easier, healthier, and authentic lives. For her, living your best life goes beyond food and fitness—it's about honoring yourself and using respect, humor, and positive reinforcement for developing strength, resiliency, and confidence.

Christine's *Right Fit* philosophy is this: if it doesn't feel good, it doesn't matter! Happiness and health can and should go hand in hand and this happens naturally when you have rhythm, regularity, and routine. Dancing, guacamole, wine, cake—nothing is off-limits as long as it's in balance with the rest of your life and goals.

A *major* '80s aficionado, Christine has also created the clothing brand *What a Feeling*, a line of wow-colored, '80s-inspired athleisure wear, customized to complement every body type. Besides looking good and feeling good, *What a Feeling* is about doing good, with a portion of every sale going to charity.

In addition to private coaching and speaking engagements, Christine can be found on Twitter and Instagram at @christinelusita, Facebook at Christine Lusita Fitness (look out for plenty of fun giveaways), and always online at www.ChristineLusita.com.

Don't forget to use the hashtag #therightfitformula, and be sure to tag Christine to connect live and share your journey with her!

Christine lives in Los Angeles, where she cannot decide whether her husband or her boxer is more adorable.

Conversion Charts

METRIC AND IMPERIAL CONVERSIONS
(These conversions are rounded for convenience)

Ingredient	Cups/Tablespoons/Teaspoons	Ounces	Grams/Milliliters
Butter	1 cup/16 tablespoons/2 sticks	8 ounces	230 grams
Cheese, shredded	1 cup	4 ounces	110 grams
Cream cheese	1 tablespoon	0.5 ounce	14.5 grams
Cornstarch	1 tablespoon	0.3 ounce	8 grams
Flour, all-purpose	1 cup/1 tablespoon	4.5 ounces/0.3 ounce	125 grams/8 grams
Flour, whole wheat	1 cup	4 ounces	120 grams
Fruit, dried	1 cup	4 ounces	120 grams
Fruits or veggies, chopped	1 cup	5 to 7 ounces	145 to 200 grams
Fruits or veggies, puréed	1 cup	8.5 ounces	245 grams
Honey, maple syrup, or corn syrup	1 tablespoon	0.75 ounce	20 grams
Liquids: cream, milk, water, or juice	1 cup	8 fluid ounces	240 milliliters
Oats	1 cup	5.5 ounces	150 grams
Salt	1 teaspoon	0.2 ounces	6 grams
Spices: cinnamon, cloves, ginger, or nutmeg (ground)	1 teaspoon	0.2 ounce	5 milliliters
Sugar, brown, firmly packed	1 cup	7 ounces	200 grams
Sugar, white	1 cup/1 tablespoon	7 ounces/0.5 ounce	200 grams/12.5 grams
Vanilla extract	1 teaspoon	0.2 ounce	4 grams

OVEN TEMPERATURES

Fahrenheit	Celsius	Gas Mark
225°	110°	¼
250°	120°	½
275°	140°	1
300°	150°	2
325°	160°	3
350°	180°	4
375°	190°	5
400°	200°	6
425°	220°	7
450°	230°	8

Index